Ketosis Guide

The Ultimate Step by Step Guide for Achieving Ketosis State & Burning Fat Rapidly

Table of Contents

Introduction

We have been told time and again how sugar makes everything better. When you're feeling down and blue, all you need is a sugar fix to get you back on your feet. And sugar truly is the body's primary source of energy. What we are told less often is that there are better energy sources. Sure, there's nothing like a bar of chocolates or a glass of sweet beverage to keep you feeling refreshed on a lousy day. The problem is after a few hours of downing the sugar, you are likely to feel out of it again. And you will be needing another fix.

Although sugar can give you energy, it is not as sustainable as you would like it to be. So, what if I told you about a much more efficient source of body fuel? It does not cause spikes of energy like sugar does. It is reliable and steady. Not many people know about it. And it rarely gets used. They are called ketones!

How do we get our bodies to produce these efficient fuel source? It's a piece of cake! We just need to break up with sugar and let our bodies get a chance to metabolize fat instead. Ketones are produced when our bodies metabolize fat. Ketones are then utilized by the cells to power themselves up and resume their normal functions.

The presence of ketones above 0.5mmol/L in the bloodstream is a metabolic state referred to as ketosis. The main objective of a ketogenic diet is to put your body in a state of ketosis. It is a way of eating prioritizing fat over carbohydrates with a moderate dose of protein. In other words, when you restrict your consumption of carbs, boost your fat intake and consume protein in moderation, you consequently assist your body into a state of ketosis.

The scientific research community has worked non-stop to understand the inner workings as well as find other potential applications of this diet called Ketogenic. More and more people are jumping into the Keto bandwagon in the hopes of losing weight.

It would be unfair though to limit the potential of the ketogenic diet to just weight loss. As a matter of fact, it can also help make a difference in overall body composition. A lot of people adopt the diet in an effort of enhancing their mood and mental performance. There is also a growing body of evidence that a ketogenic diet has therapeutic benefits and is also capable of disease prevention.

So if the ketogenic diet is that great, why haven't you heard of it before? I can think of one major reason and that is you have been brainwashed into thinking that calorie counting is the best way to lose weight ever! Or you still cling onto the lie that sugar defines life. But if you are ready to try a much better way of staying healthy and keeping in great shape, I invite you to explore ketosis through the ketogenic diet with me.

Chapter 1 - The Ketosis State: Why You Want It?

Before we go into details about this much desired metabolic state called ketosis, let's go back to the basics first. This will help you better understand why ketosis is important and why you would want to be a part of it.

The Food Process

Our bodies rely on what we feed it. On an average day when you're having bagel, pasta or sandwich for lunch with unlimited dessert, your body's cells utilize glucose as the primary energy source. As you know, glucose comes from dietary carbohydrates. It's in sugar. No, we're not just talking about what you put in your coffee. There's also sugar in fruits, yogurt, milk, beverages and pretty much almost every packaged food. Dietary carbohydrates also include starchy foods which can be found in pasta, bread, etc. Can you think of a day when you're not feasting on dietary carbohydrates?

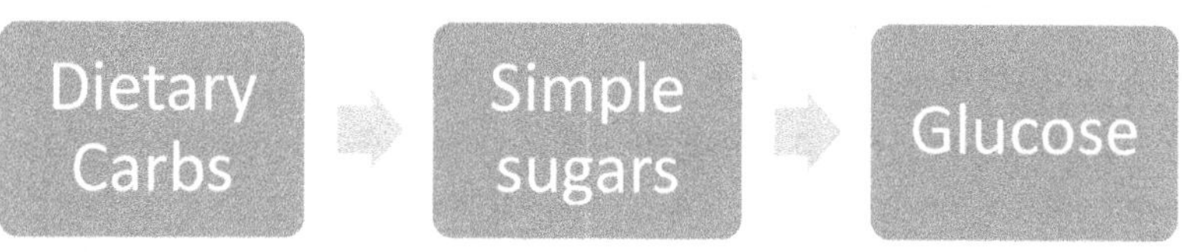

This is how it works. Dietary carbohydrates are essentially simple sugars which the body breaks down and turns into glucose. To function, your body obtains energy from the glucose it produced as a result of what you consumed. The problem is, not all of this new glucose supply gets to be used as energy. The body is clever and it is especially adept at saving.

So what remains of the glucose is stored as fat. And this my friend, is how we gain weight.

Burning and Storing Sugar

Do you know how much sugar is in a blueberry muffin? It contains 100 grams of sugar. Now a calorie counting method will tell you that 1 gram of sugar is equivalent to 4 calories. That's 400 calories from a blueberry muffin which you can burn through exercise. In truth, the process is much more complicated than this.

Burning Through Physical Exercise

Not all of these sugar gets processed to be used as body fuel. Did you know that for every gram of sugar, .06 gram gets automatically stored as fat? That means for every blueberry muffin your body automatically stores 6 grams which contribute to body fat storage. For every gram of sugar, only 50 percent becomes available for energy. Moreover, there is no guarantee that running can burn 50 grams of sugar.

You see burning depends on weight too. 30 minutes of running will have a different impact on a 240-pound man versus a 125-pound woman. Generally, more energy is required to move a larger body. In which case, those who weigh much more tend to burn more calories for every hour of any type of activity. So, a smaller body will have to work twice as hard to burn the same amount as a larger person. This is why as people begin to lose weight, they can't simply rely on the same diet and training program and still expect to lose some more on the same rate. As the body gets lighter, the amount of exercise necessary for weight loss increases.

If you want to burn more, you have to take on more vigorous exercises. Let's talk on a language most people understand. That is burning calories. If you're 125 pounds who wants to burn 400 calories, you will need a 45-minutes worth of high impact step aerobics. That is also equivalent to one hour of high impact regular aerobics or low impact step aerobics. If you're 155 pounds, you require 30 minutes on high-intensity stationary bike. The same amount of time spent on a low impact regular aerobics will only burn half of 400 calories. At 185 pounds, you will need to spend half an hour on the elliptical machine. And at 200 pounds, you will only need half an hour on the stair treadmill to burn off the same amount of 400 calories.

Sport is also an excellent form of exercise. For a 125-pound individual, an hour spent playing tennis or soccer, ice skating or rollerblading can burn over 400 calories. Running for half an hour at 8.6 mph can achieve the same goal. A 155-pound individual, on the other hand, will only need half an hour swimming or rock climbing to burn 400 calories. For a 185-pound individual, it will take half an hour cross country running or sparring to burn over 400 calories.

Doing chores can also help burn excess baggage but it will take a combination of activities. For instance, an individual who weighs 185 pounds needs 30 minutes cooking and another 30 minutes carrying boxes to burn 400 calories. A 155-pound individual will have to spend 30 minutes in rearranging furniture and another 30 minutes playing with children to burn the same amount of calories. Meanwhile, an hour raking the lawn and half an hour chopping wood will help a 125-pound individual can maximize the burning.

What if you are not the sporty type? What if you don't have the patience or the time to go to the gym? Or what if you simply don't like the idea of sweating it out, do you have a chance of losing weight? What are your options?

Getting in shape means making an effort to become physically active. A sedentary lifestyle contributes significantly to the epidemic that is obesity. Exercise can make a difference. However, if you're attempting to lose some weight, you can probably get a good start by making a change in your diet. And that's our starting point in this book.

Cut Off the Sugar

Burning sugar requires quite an exercise. If you can't commit to training, you should definitely think about cutting off sugar from your diet. The body gets used to processing carbs and breaking them down to simple sugar so when you deprive it of that supply, it will try to look for another source of fuel.

When the energy demands of the body are not met by enough glucose, it will naturally adapt and find another way to meet the needs. This is when the body begins to process and break down fat to meet energy demands. This is ketosis.

Chapter 2 - Ketosis and the History of Humans

Because we have become used to burning carbohydrates and relying on sugar for energy, we don't realize that given the chance, the body would prefer to burn ketones for energy. I've mentioned earlier that it takes a lot for the body to enter ketosis. And that is mainly because of the diet we are used to.

Human history will tell us, however, that ketone burning was actually necessary for survival. Our ancestors did not have food delivery hotlines, frozen foods or refrigerators for that matter, supermarkets and convenient stores. Food was not readily available to them. If they want to have a meal, it will take more than swiping their cards. They had to hunt for food, meal after meal, throughout the year and their lifetime. Unfortunately, there were days when they feasted and there were days or weeks when they had none.

Needless to say, the food environment where our ancestors lived in was unpredictable. Because of this, their bodies adapted to the circumstances. Food scarcity is inevitable. In which case, their bodies had to rely on different sources of energy. For instance, stored glycogen was useful in keeping them energized in times when there was nothing to eat. Stored fat was also useful in providing them a more sustained fuel source to help them last for extended periods of time without food.

In principle, fat and glycogen are enough to keep the body functioning for extended periods of time with food scarcity. The brain is another matter, however. Fatty acids can keep the rest of the human system functioning but the brain cells require a more specialized fuel. Fatty acids are not that reliable because they are rather too slow to process. Plus, they also tend to produce reactive oxygen species as a result of being processed and burned. This leaves the brain cells in a vulnerable position. They become at risk of starvation and damage.

BUT like we mentioned previously, the human bodily system is smart. To protect the brain from damage and starvation, the liver processes amino acids from protein and other non-sugar substrates and converts them into sugar. This is a process known as gluconeogenesis. Thanks to gluconeogenesis, the brain is saved. Yay to the liver!

There is one problem, however. Although the process of gluconeogenesis can help the brain continue to function, it is not able to prevent muscle loss. According to health and fitness expert from the University of Connecticut, Dr. Chris Masterjohn, to meet the energy demands of the brain during periods of fasting, about 2.2 pounds of lean muscle mass will have to be converted into sugar every single day. If this is the case, the body can easily and quickly burn through muscle and there won't be enough left to fuel and energize it for a food-finding mission.

So how come our ancestors survived and thrived instead of withering away like flies? They may have been unlucky in the unpredictable food environment thing but they were fortunate to have ketosis.

The bottom line is our bodies have naturally evolved with the ability to process and burn ketones for energy as a way of powering the brain while preserving muscle mass.

What is Gluconeogenesis?

The liver has many responsibilities and one of which is gluconeogenesis. It is a process performed by the liver to keep the level of blood sugar constant. The liver depends on peptide hormones, insulin and glucagon to regulate gluconeogenesis.

When we consume an insulin-stimulating meal like breakfast cereal, for instance, the pancreas is prompted to secrete insulin. In response, the cells will begin to process and burn sugar. As insulin reaches the liver and interacts with the liver cells, it works to inhibit the process of gluconeogenesis and encourages the storage of glycogen.

Once the cells in the body have burned the sugar, insulin and blood sugar levels begin to drop. The pancreas responds by releasing glucagon. As the glucagon level increases, the liver is stimulated and will begin the process of breaking stored glycogen down. This will encourage gluconeogenesis to start providing sugar to the cells. At the same time, the fat cells release fatty acids supply into the blood.

Without a carb intake, the liver will keep on breaking glycogen down and utilize the process of gluconeogenesis in an effort to provide energy to the body. How long will the glycogen storage last? The depletion of glycogen storage may begin between 6 and 24 hours of restricting carb intake. The body will then switch to relying on gluconeogenesis as the primary source of energy. At this stage, muscle loss can begin. The body will start burning through muscle mass at a quick pace if it doesn't receive sufficient calories.

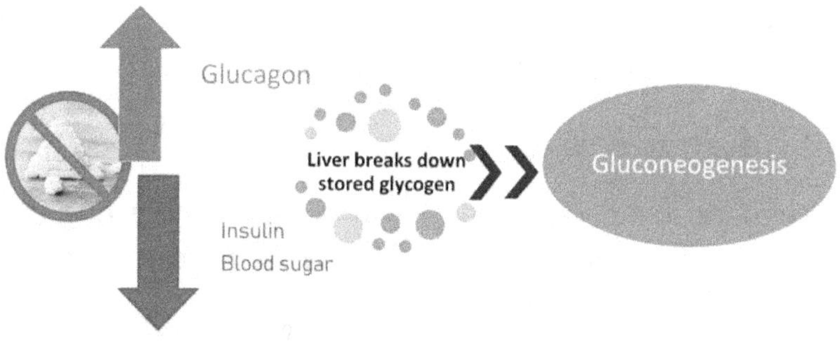

Gluconeogenesis is an expensive process. It requires a lot of energy. As the liver cells continue to be deprived, it will eventually run out of energy to spend on the process. To resolve the situation, these liver cells will turn on ketogenic amino acids and fatty acids. They will be converted to ketones for energy supply. At this point, the body just joined the ketosis party!

How long does it take for the liver to start rounding up and jumpstarting ketone production?

Forgive me for saying this but it depends on each individual. The answer is more complex. Generally, the process takes much longer for people who barely exercise. It's the same case for fasting virgins and those who are used to having carbs every meal. It will take much longer for them to elevate ketone production and graduate from gluconeogenesis.

Men are also included in this bracket. Their bodies require more time to enter ketosis. Heavy reliance on gluconeogenesis without stepping into ketosis can occur. Usually, it will take 1 to about 9 days after glycogen supply is depleted.

The safe answer is to endure carb restriction for 2 or up to 10 days. That is the usual deadline for the liver to acquaint itself to the metabolic process of ketogenesis to level up the production of ketones for fuel and advance to ketosis.

What is Ketogenesis?

Let's expand our vocabulary further by learning about ketogenesis also known as the metabolic process behind the metabolic state called ketosis.

Confused? Let's have a little playback. Ketosis is the metabolic state your body is at when the ketones levels in your blood reach a certain point. Your body doesn't reach this state with fairy dust. The body makes it possible by going through a biochemical process that is called ketogenesis.

The mitochondria in the liver cells are mainly responsible for this process. Ketogenesis continuously occurs but only to a minimal degree. The liver cells use this process to continue to provide ketone to fuel the renal cortex of the kidney and the heart.

When glycogen runs out and the liver can't deliver sufficient energy for the entire body through gluconeogenesis, it begins to rely on ketogenesis in order to produce ketones to feed the heart, the muscles, and the brain cells.

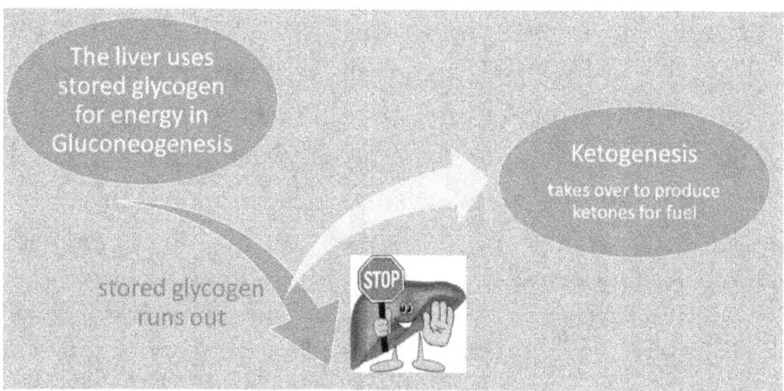

During ketogenesis, amino acids such as leucine and lysine and fatty acids are turned into ketone body acetoacetate which is in turn, converted to either acetone or beta-hydroxybutyrate (BHB).

Acetone is a ketone body and they are the least abundant. However, under special circumstances, their production increases to higher quantities. This usually occurs when you begin following a ketogenic diet.

Keto Adaptation

The cells begin to adapt as you continue with carbohydrate restriction. At this stage, BHB becomes the predominant ketone body. The muscle cells and the brain begin to rely on it as the primary fuel. This is called keto-adaptation.

After some weeks of entering and staying in ketosis, your body becomes keto-adapted. At this level, ketones provide about 70 percent of the brain's energy requirements and supply as much as 50 percent of basal energy needs. In other words, at this point, your body meets the following benefits.

-Preserve your muscle mass

-Power the brain

-Burn ketones for energy

Remember the mitochondria in liver cells? They are the superhero of ketogenesis. During keto-adaptation, more of them emerge in the ketone burning cells. And the already existing ones become much more efficient in their job of assisting with ketone metabolism. Imagine Ironman getting an upgrade and getting more help from his Avenger friends! That's what happens here.

So what happens when the Avenger gang of mitochondria work together? Ketone burning cells get an upgrade. This also makes it easier for your body to return to ketosis after reintroducing carbohydrates back to your diet.

We've talked about how long it usually takes for all this magic to happen. There are two routes to ketogenesis and keto-adaptation.

1. Fasting and intense exercise
2. Ketogenic diet

You can do it the way our hunter-gatherer ancestors have done it. Remember their story of not being able to feed for days and weeks at a time or the way they manage to go out full force hunting? In the modern world, we know this as fasting and intense exercise. This is probably the quickest route to reaching ketosis and keto-adaptation. However, it is neither the healthiest nor the most sustainable way to maintain ketosis.

Alright. So our ancestors were able to do it, why can't we? Unlike them, we simply are not used to long fasting anymore. The availability of food ruined that for us.

The longer but smarter move is to take the second route. Keto-adaptation has plenty of benefits to offer. To maximize that without putting our physical function and health at risk, what I recommend is to stick with a ketogenic diet.

Fasting can undoubtedly stimulate the metabolic processes we've talked about. The ketogenic diet, however, can work just as well as fasting in stimulating these processes. What makes the ketogenic diet effective?

One of the main things about this diet is the way it encourages the restriction of carbohydrates. By doing so, your insulin levels and blood sugar drop. As a result of this, your glucagon levels elevate and your body is prompted to burn glycogen and produce more ketones.

What about protein? When you eat a protein-rich food, your insulin levels also increase. However, moderate consumption of protein will not stop you from entering ketosis. The only downside to the ketogenic diet is that it won't get to a ketosis state as quickly as fasting would. In a ketogenic diet, you are encouraged to consume fat and moderate protein while limiting your carb consumption. Your body won't be starved but the diet is also the safer way to go.

If protein can also increase insulin levels, what's the use of keeping it in the diet? The shortest way is not always the best way. Muscle loss is a big issue in fasting. It may not occur in a 24 to 48 hour fast but it will eventually happen. Protein plays an important role in the preservation of muscle mass. It also helps the body maintain physical performance. And this is a big deal in a ketogenic diet.

According to research studies, ketogenic dieters who limited their protein intake to 1.2 grams or less per kilogram of their body weight are more likely to experience a dreaded progressive loss of their lean muscle tissue. It also impaired their physical performance.

Ketogenic dieters who maintained 1.5 grams intake of protein per kilogram of their body weight, however, were successfully able to maintain their ability to perform physically. It also allowed them to keep their muscle mass intact.

While too little protein consumption is not advisable, too much is also counterproductive. When you have too much protein in a ketogenic diet, you run the risk of suppressing ketogenesis. As a result, you will experience ketosis at a lower level. So how much exactly is too much and how little is too low?

The recommendation is to dedicate 15 percent to 25 percent of your daily calorie intake to protein. This will ensure a deep level of ketosis and at the same time maintain physical function and muscle mass.

The recommendation will vary if you do weightlifting or follow a high-intensity workout on a regular basis. In this case, your body will be able to sustain a deep level of ketosis even if you slightly increase your protein consumption than the recommendation above.

Chapter 3 - Keto Diet versus Calorie Counting

The Ketogenic diet and calorie counting both work toward the same goal, weight loss. They are very different in approach however. While Keto suggests a list of unacceptable and acceptable foods, no such list exists in a calorie counting approach. What matters is the number.

The Calorie Counting Approach

In this weight loss method, the numbers in everything you drink and eat matters. The only rule is to consume fewer calories than what your body can actually burn. The challenge is in making the calculations right. You will need to count the number of calories your body requires in order to keep at your current weight. The calculation looks something like this.

For instance, a person who weighs 150 pounds will require 2,250 daily calorie intake to keep at 150. Depending on your goal, you shall subtract the amount of calories from the 2,250 recommended daily intake. For example, your goal is to lose 1

to 2 pounds a week, you will then take away around 500 to 1,000 from your daily maintenance calories. Based on the example above, you will end up with 1,250 to 1,750 daily calorie goal.

Because calorie counting has become so popular, the computation has been made easy. Most food items note their calorie content in their packaging. There are even apps available to help people keep track of their calorie intake. This is one of the major selling points of the calorie counting approach. It's quite simple to do.

With the calorie counting approach, there is no need to make a drastic change in the way you eat. There are no specific restrictions on what you should and should not indulge in. There is, however, a general recommendation to fill your daily calorie needs with more nutritious foods like whole grains, nuts, fruits, beans, vegetables, lean protein, etc. Most diets that follow the calorie counting approach also recommend choosing the non-fat or low-fat food options.

The idea of calorie counting does sound sensible enough. And it has worked for some people. The flaw in the calorie counting approach is the way it assumes that all calories are equal. Are they?

Are All Calories Equal?

This is a subject matter that is debated in the scientific circle. Do you remember the law of conservation of energy? According to this law, energy can neither be created nor destroyed. If we apply this law to the maintenance of weight, we can come up with this very basic formula.

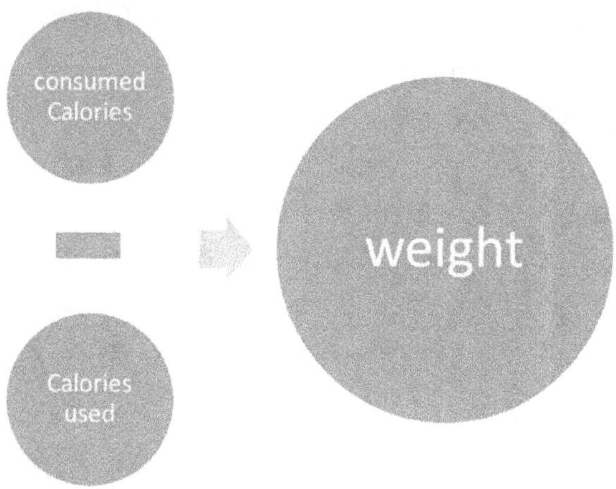

This point of view implies that where you get the calories from is not important. The type of food you put in your mouth does not matter. As long as it is calorie, it counts. All calories are treated equally. So in order to lose weight, you need to have a calorie deficit. This can be done by either burning more from what your calorie intake or reducing your calorie consumption.

Keto agrees that calories do count. However, it also puts an emphasis on the kind of consumed those calories are obtained from. The food type does have an impact on the amount of energy needed to process, burn and use it. Certain food types will take more energy to burn than others. There are also types of food that are likely to cause cravings.

Let's take the case of carbohydrates versus protein. The body finds it easiest to process and store carbs than any other food types. Protein, on the other hand, is a bit more of a challenge for the body because it requires more energy to burn or store it. This is referred to as the thermic effect. And there are several studies to prove it.

One of which found that more energy is spent by individuals who took high protein versus high carb, low-fat meals (Johnston, Day, & Swan, 2002). In another study, the researchers focused on diets according to their macronutrient composition and their effect on the amount of energy expenditure. A reduced resting energy expenditure is caused by weight loss. This is more commonly known as metabolic rate. When the metabolic rate goes down, weight regain becomes more likely to occur. According to the results of the study, a high protein and restricted carb diet caused the least effect on decreasing resting energy expenditure during weight loss (Ebbeling et al, 2012).

The second law of thermodynamics states that there is always a loss of some energy in any chemical reaction. It supports the idea of the thermic effect that some food possesses. Thermic effect simply means that energy will be expended as heat. In this case, not all calories are equal (Feinman & Fine, 2004).

If we are being more accurate about it, the amount of energy expended is affected by three factors: physical activity, resting metabolic rate and thermic effect. 32 percent of calories in are spent through physical activity and 8 percent energy loss is caused by the thermic effect. The biggest cut goes to resting metabolic rate at 60 percent. In other words, the type of calories matters more than you're used to paying attention to.

There are other factors that affect the equation. For instance, different kinds of food also affect hormonal changes. High carb diets are known to increase insulin levels. This important to note because higher insulin levels also mean higher fat storage. On the other hand, low insulin levels can promote the burning of fat. A lower insulin level will make the body want to burn rather than store fat.

Yes, weight loss can be achieved if you burn more calories than the amount you consume. However, it is also important to note the macronutrient composition of these calories. Different foods affect the body to a varying degree. While some can speed up the metabolic rate, other tend to slow it down. Different foods also cause hormonal effects on your body. Whether those effects are favorable or unfavorable for weight loss, depends on the food you choose.

In this case, counting is not all that matters. It is incredibly important to choose where your calories are coming from. As such will affect the way your body processes it, whether they are burned more efficiently or stored.

By now you understand why protein should be on a higher level than carbohydrates in your food pyramid. But what about fat?

Fat for Fat Loss?

To lose weight, you need to watch out for fat. This has been drilled into our brains. And this is why most of us make an effort to select non-fat and low-fat food options. To explain why this is all a lie

Researchers conducted a review involving 13 randomized controlled trials. According to their findings, a keto diet allowed the patients to lose a significant amount of weight, much more than those who were on low-fat diets. They were also able to keep the weight off for about 12 months or even more (Bueno, de Melo, de Oliveira, & da Rocha, 2013).

In another review, 17 randomized controlled trials were involved. Researchers found that patients lost more weight using a low carb diet compared to a low-fat diet (Sackner-Bernstein, Kanter, & Kaul, 2015). Another study found that type 2 diabetes patients also benefit significantly from a diet-induced ketosis. Results showed that patients had lost 12 percent of their body weight after following the diet for a year (Hallberg et al, 2018).

There's an argument that the weight loss experienced by people following a low carb diet is predominantly water weight. And yes, water loss occurs when glycogen supply is depleted. However, studies also prove that weight loss achieved through a keto diet that lasts for a few weeks or more is predominantly fat rather than water weight (Volek et al, 2002).

The Major Differences between Keto Diet and Calorie Counting

Based on all the arguments we've made above and the supporting evidence, there is no doubt that following a ketogenic diet is way more effective for weight loss than a calorie counting approach. There are two major reasons for these and they are the following.

-Keto diet has the metabolic advantage.

-Keto diet promotes appetite suppression.

The Metabolic Advantage of Keto

Two persons can consume the same amount of calories but their weight loss won't be equal. Let's say you and your friend consumes 1500 calories a day. Your 1500 calories come from high fat and protein, low carb while your friend's diet consists of high carb low-fat one. Chances are, you will become more successful in attaining your weight loss goal.

The distinct advantage of a low carb diet comes from the increased amount of energy expended. Your diet allows your body to burn calories at a higher rate. This can be attributed to two factors: thermic effect and fat burning.

We've mentioned protein earlier and its thermic effect. When you focus on protein more than you do carbs, it will cost you more energy to burn it. As you restrict your carb consumption, your body makes use of protein to produce glucose. This is the process referred to as gluconeogenesis. But how much energy exactly will be spent by the thermic effect of protein? The estimated energy cost is somewhere between ~400 and 600 calories a day (Paoli, Rubini, Volek, & Grimaldi, 2013). This only comes as a result of changing the food you eat, from high carb to low carb and more protein focused.

Keto diet also increases your body's ability to burn fat. During the keto-adaptation phase, your body is able to increase the fat burning rate twice as much. This is an achievement that a high carb diet can only dream of. But that is not all. As insulin levels decrease, the body is also prompted to not only increase fat burning but also decrease fat storage as well as elevate lean muscle mass (Feinman & Fine, 2007).

Appetite Suppression through Keto

You may hardly feel the thermic effect of food or the increased fat burning rate so let's make it more real. Let's jump into an issue that dieters usually face, hunger!

A systematic review of the ketogenic diet revealed appetite suppression as one of its common symptoms (Gibson et al, 2015). But how does this happen? It comes as a result of nutritional ketosis which can also be linked to the change in diet. You see, protein and fat, unlike carbs, can make you feel full for a longer period of time. By restricting carbs and increasing the consumption of fat and protein instead, you are able to avoid the most dreaded factor of dieting, that hungry feeling.

Also, in a state of ketosis, the hormone that increases the feeling of hunger ghrelin is suppressed (Sumithran et al, 2013). We've talked about the ketone BHB earlier. This ketone body also serves as a satiety signal (Johnstone, Horgan, Murison, Bremner, & Lobley, 2008). The more of this the body produces during ketosis, the less likely you'll be bothered by your appetite.

It's simpler to think of higher expenditure of energy and appetite suppression as independent players. But the truth is they are likely to work hand in hand. For instance, with an increased consumption of protein rather than carbs, more energy is expended and body temperature increases. This event can also translate to emulating the feeling of fullness.

Doesn't the same thing happen when you're counting calories?

This is a sensible question. The answer to it is a big NO. As a matter of fact, calorie restricted diets tend to work in a completely opposite way.

Counting calories is much easier to do but have you ever wondered why people who get into these calorie restricted diets usually fail? The main reason for yo-yo dieting is the uncontrollable hunger that comes as a result of cutting calories. While restricting your calorie intake can no doubt, help you lose weight, it is less likely a sustainable one. It changes your hormones alright but instead of helping you control your appetite like a ketogenic diet does, calorie restriction approach makes your hormones to drive you to feel even more hungry.

Carbs create a vicious cycle of hunger. As long as you keep feeding on more carbs, you're stuck in the cycle. This is why keto encourages you to break away from it.

Chapter 4 - Benefits of Ketosis

The Ketogenic diet has been receiving a lot of attention in the scientific circle and the weight loss arena. On one hand are those that believe it to be the best diet ever! On the other are those who are extremely doubtful.

In truth, the keto diet is more than just another weight loss fad diet. It is unfair to limit its benefits to weight loss.

A solid body of scientific evidence proves that this diet can significantly benefit people with certain conditions including the following.

- Migraines
- Fatty Liver Disease
- Polycystic Ovary Syndrome
- Heart Disease
- Obesity
- High Blood Sugar Levels
- Chronic Inflammation
- Parkinson's Disease
- Alzheimer's Disease
- High Blood Pressure
- Type 1 and Type 2 Diabetes
- Epilepsy
- Cancer

It does not promise to magically cure people suffering from these conditions but it may be able to help improve their circumstances.

Whether or not you are at risk of any of the above conditions, you can still benefit from following a keto diet for the following reasons.

- Keto can promote better brain function.
- It can help in reducing inflammation.
- Keto boosts energy level.
- It helps in improving your body composition.

More than Calories

Some researchers argue that the main reason for the benefits of keto is the way it makes individuals consume fewer calories on the diet. According to this argument, ketone burning for fuel and the carb restriction takes the back seat.

Yes, ketogenic diet prompts people to consume fewer calories thanks to the satiating effect of high fat and moderate protein meals. And yes as a result of lesser calorie intake, people experience weight loss and improved overall health. To put calories at the center of the equation, however, is limiting. This argument fails to consider a lot of more important things that go on inside the body during ketosis.

We've talked about how a keto diet works to elicit important bodily mechanisms. Most of these mechanisms do not occur in other diets. The unique mechanisms prompted by the keto diet explains its many important benefits, mechanisms that simply cannot be explained by limiting ourselves to the calorie perspective.

Keto Works on a Cellular Level

We've already mentioned how the body plays favorites when it comes to using carbohydrates as the primary fuel source. Cut the carbs and the body responds as if it's under fasting. But the body won't simply give up, it requires energy to function so it looks for another fuel source. As a result, new energy pathways are stimulated to meet the energy requirements of the cells. Among these pathways is ketogenesis. And through ketogenesis, an alternative fuel comes into play, the ketone body. Every cell in the body now makes use of these ketone bodies for fuel with the exception of red blood cells and liver.

Keto Changes the Body

From the body's perspective, keto's effects begin when insulin levels are changed. Carbs are known as the biggest factor that stimulates insulin. Take carbs out of the equation and insulin levels go down, fat burning activity is elevated and inflammation is reduced. Chronic diseases are driven by three major drivers. These are insulin resistance, fat accumulation, and inflammation. Changes enforced by keto in the body effectively address these primary drivers which can possibly save you from chronic diseases.

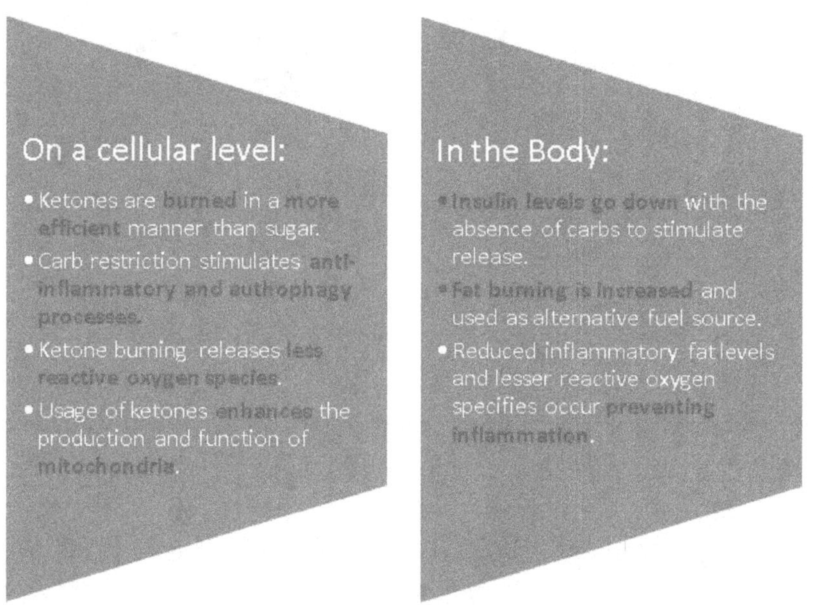

Keto helps in treating epilepsy

The ketogenic diet did not exactly start out as a diet specifically formulated for weight loss. It was begun in 1924 by Dr. Russell Wilder as a carb restricted diet. The main objective was to assist in the treatment of epilepsy in children.

Epilepsy is characterized by unpredictable and recurrent seizures. The seizures result from abnormal activities in the brain. It is a nervous system disorder.

In a study published in 1998 involved 150 epileptic children. Most of these patients experienced seizures twice a week even after taking a minimum of two medications specific for seizures. After 3 months of following a ketogenic diet, 34 percent of the children experienced more than 90 percent reduction in seizures.

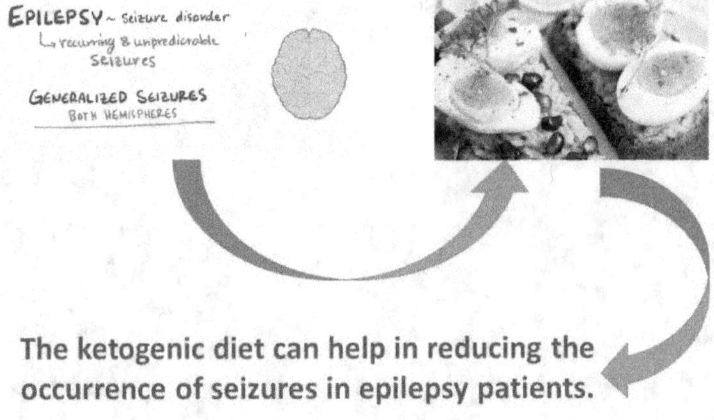

The ketogenic diet can help in reducing the occurrence of seizures in epilepsy patients.

After 6 months, 71 percent stayed on the diet and 32 percent of whom had more than 90 percent seizure reduction. After a whole year, 55 percent remained on a ketogenic diet and 37 percent of whom experienced 90 percent decrease in seizures.

The researchers concluded that ketogenic diet did not only help these children by reducing their seizure episodes. The diet was actually more helpful as anticonvulsant compared to some of the most commonly used drugs for epilepsy (Freeman et al, 1998).

The Lancet Journal of Neurology published a meta-analysis of 19 studies involving 1084 patients. It was focused on evaluating the effect of the diet in the treatment of epilepsy. The conclusion was that patients who remained on the diet increased their treatment success by 2.25 times. In terms of seizure reduction, that amounts to at least 50 percent (Neal et al, 2008).

Ketogenic diet may help in the reversal of Type 2 diabetes.

Insulin resistance is an issue that should not be taken lightly. It usually leads to prediabetes which, if not managed properly, can lead to type 2 diabetes. A change in lifestyle and diet is necessary and this is where the ketogenic diet comes in. because it promotes a low carb intake, people who follow the diet can reduce their insulin levels until it reaches a healthy level. It can also help in reversing insulin resistance.

Researchers from the Duke University Medical Center conducted a ketogenic diet intervention trial among type 2 diabetes patients for 16 weeks. The subjects followed a ketogenic diet consuming below 20 grams of carbs a day. At the same time, their diabetes medication was reduced. At the end of the trial, researchers observed that the subjects had a 16 percent decrease in their Hemoglobin Ac. The patients' body weight also decreased by 8.7 kg. Also, their blood glucose levels were reduced at an average of 16.6 percent. There was also a decrease in their triglyceride levels at an average of 41.6 percent (Yancy et al, 2005).

By the end of the trial, most of the subjects either reduced or discontinued their medications. In conclusion, the researchers stated that a low carb ketogenic diet is effective in lowering blood glucose. They advise that in order to ensure the most favorable outcome, type 2 diabetes patients should consult with their doctor before applying any adjustments to their diabetes medication (Yancy et al, 2005).

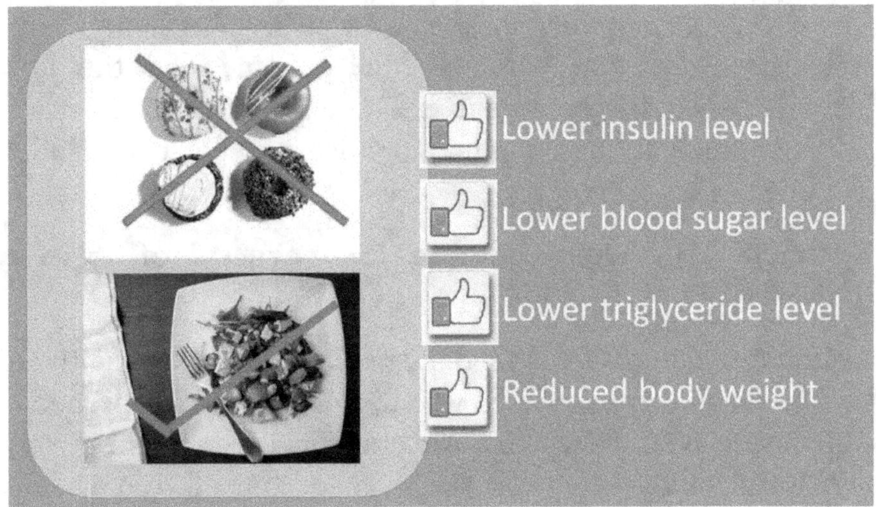

Even if you are not pre-diabetic or suffering from type 2 diabetes, you can benefit from this diet. Studies show that similar improvements can be experienced by healthy individuals.

Keto Can Help in Controlling Type 1 Diabetes.

Both Type 1 and Type 2 diabetes patients suffer from blood sugar issues. However, while type 2 diabetes patients are insulin resistant, type 1 diabetes patients have an inability of producing enough insulin or they are unable to produce any insulin at all. This is why they require insulin administration. The ketogenic diet may not be able to help in reversing this condition but it can help in managing the disease. Research shows that a low carb whole foods based diet is best in controlling type 1 diabetes (Tóth & Clemens, 2014).

Keto Can Help Keep Blood Pressure Level Healthy.

High blood pressure is the cause of around 12.8 percent of deaths according to the World Health Organization. A drastic change in lifestyle and diet is essential in correcting this condition. The ketogenic diet, in particular, can prove helpful in managing high blood pressure and keeping it at a healthy level.

In a 2007 study, researchers conducted a 12-month trial to assess four diets including low carb diet and their effects on blood pressure and cardiovascular fitness. All of the diets showed improvements in the subjects' LDL cholesterol, triglycerides, and body mass. The low carb subjects, however, achieved the best results (Gardner et al, 2007).

In another study, researchers compared low carb diet to a low-fat diet. In the low-fat diet, the participants were even given Orlistat, medication for weight loss and lowering blood pressure. At the end of the study, the researchers concluded that participants on the low carb dietary invention showed better results. It was clearly more effective for keeping blood pressure low (Yancy et al, 2010).

Keto Can Help Improve the Condition of Alzheimer Patients.

You now know that sugar is bad news for the brain. As a matter of fact, a scientific review revealed that high carb consumption can even make the behavior and cognitive performance of Alzheimer patients worse. So how does a ketogenic diet fare on this brain function thing?

According to scientific evidence, keto can actually help and possibly reverse Alzheimer's. Remember the ketone body

BHB? In a research experiment, ketone supplementation with BHB was found to improve the memory function of people suffering from the disease. Other scientists back up these findings.

In one study, researchers administered MCT oil to Alzheimer patients before testing their memory. After being given MCT oil, the patients showed a better number of ketone bodies in their blood levels. And when they were tested, they showed greater memory recall (Henderson et al, 2009).

Keto Can Reduce the Symptoms of Parkinson's Disease.

Parkinson's disease is characterized by abnormalities in movement, cognition, and cortical functions. Because ketone bodies may be able to bypass mitochondrial complex defects, it may be able to help PD patients as well. In a small clinical study, 5 out of 7 patients reported having improved their scores on a PD rating scale (Vanitallie et al., 2005).

An in vitro experiment published in the Journal of Neurochemistry demonstrated the same protective effects of ketone bodies against cognitive impairment and mitochondrial dysfunction (Kim et al, 2010). Other scientists hypothesize that the improvement in symptoms experienced by PD patients following a ketogenic diet may be attributed to the increased consumption of essential fatty acids.

Keto Can Assist in the Improvement of Cholesterol Levels and in Reversing Heart Diseases.

The main reason why a lot of people make great efforts in looking for non- or low-fat options is the idea that fat increases cholesterol. Yes, ketogenic diet is high in saturated fat but contrary to the common belief, the diet can actually improve rather than hurt your cholesterol levels. Not only that, keto has also been found to be helpful in reducing the risk of heart disease. Science also backs this up.

Before we go science-sy on this, let's make a few things clear. Cholesterol is not all bad. While LDL cholesterol is mainly bad, HDL cholesterol is actually good. For heart health, you would want to keep your LDL low and your HDL high at a healthy level.

In a meta-analysis including 12 studies where 1257 patients were examined, researchers assessed the effects of a very low carb ketogenic diet based on cardiovascular health key metrics which includes HDL cholesterol. In this diet, the researchers defined very low cholesterol as less than 50g of carbs a day. They also compared the impact of VLCKD on low-fat diets.

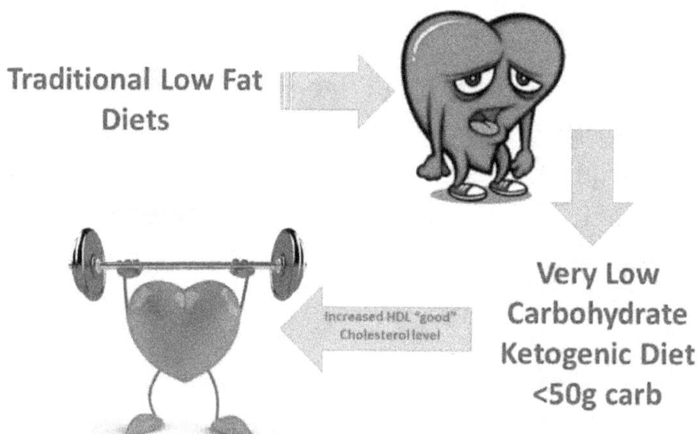

In their assessment, they found that patients who went under VLCKD showed an average increase in their HDL level at 0.12 mmol/L which was twice more than the HDL 0.06 mmol/L recorded in patients who followed low-fat diets. Because of the significant improvement in HDL levels, the researchers concluded that the carb-restricted diet proves to offer cardiovascular benefits (Bueno et al, 2013). Several studies also found that carb restricted diets are effective in decreasing LDL and VLDL particles which reduces cardiovascular disease risks.

Keto Can Potentially Treat Polycystic Ovary Syndrome and Infertility.

PCOS or Polycystic Ovary Syndrome is one of the major causes of infertility in women. In fact, 70 percent of female infertility issues are caused by this syndrome. But what causes PCOS?

High insulin levels are to be blamed. High levels of insulin drive the ovaries to produce more of testosterone-like androgens and at the same time, reduce the production of globulin. Globulin is responsible for preventing testosterone from entering the cells freely.

If there are more androgens and not much globulin, there's nothing to stop testosterone from interacting with the cells and floating through blood. For women, this is a nightmare. It can cause anything from abnormal facial or chest hair growth, acne, fatigue, mood swings and low sex drive. The most devastating issues this situation creates are infertility and a variety of other PCOS symptoms. If insulin levels remain high or even continue to increase, PCOS symptoms can get much worse.

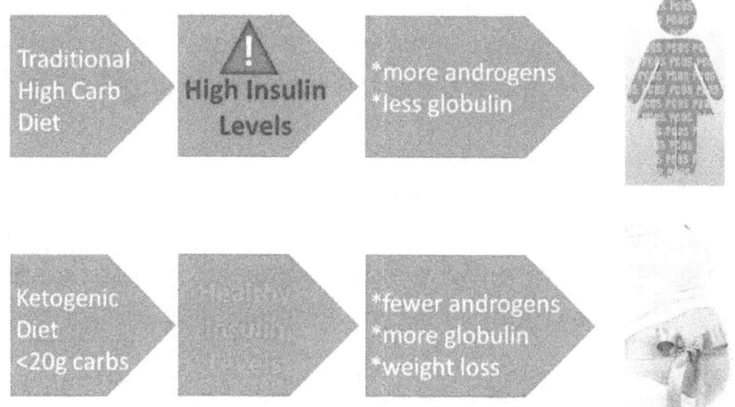

One study assessed the impact of ketogenic diet in women suffering from PCOS. For 24 weeks, the female subjects followed a ketogenic diet consisting of 20 grams or fewer carbohydrates in a day. The subjects experienced weight loss in an average of 12 percent. The more impressive result is that they recorded a reduction in free testosterone by 22 percent. Their insulin levels were significantly reduced by 54 percent. The most astounding of all is that two of the women from the study actually got pregnant despite facing infertility issues before the study (Mavropoulos, Yancy, Hepburn, & Westman, 2005).

Ketogenic Diet Can Help in Preventing and Reducing the Severity of Headaches and Migraines.

Ketone bodies can work against migraines because of their ability to inhibit neural inflammation and at the same time, improve the brain mitochondrial metabolism. Ketone bodies also reduce oxidative stress and block high concentrations of glutamate which are present in epilepsy and migraine sufferers.

A review of the impact of ketogenic diet on migraines revealed that the diet treats headaches and reduces the need for medication in migraine sufferers. On the other hand, scientists found that a standard low-calorie diet was completely ineffective in treating migraine (Di Lorenzo, Coppola, Sirianni, & Pierelli, 2013).

To sum it all up, the ketogenic diet can assist in either reversing or reducing the symptoms of health conditions. While it is definitely not a magical panacea, scientific studies prove that the keto diet can serve the interest of a lot of people.

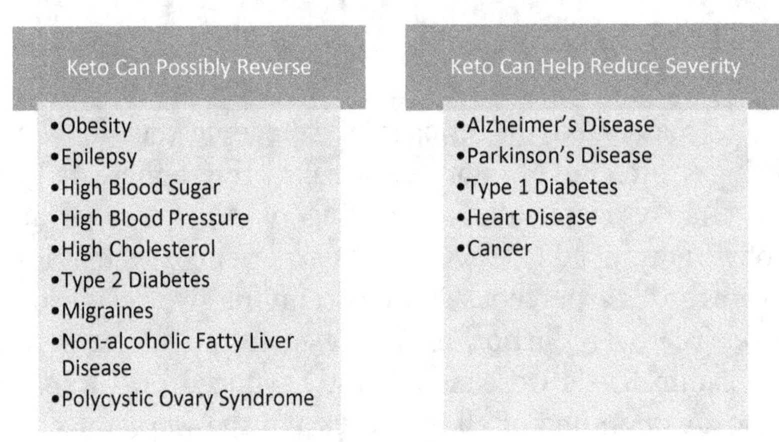

What if you're generally healthy and you could care less about the above mentioned health conditions? There's no need to create a problem to be solved by the ketogenic diet. The exciting thing about this diet is that it is generally suited for everyone.

You can boost your brain function.

If you're on a ketogenic diet, you can expect your brain to work more properly. With keto comes more efficient brain cells. Through keto, inflammation in the brain is reduced and neurotrophic factors that promote health are activated. These benefits come as a result of the combined forces of ketone bodies and restricted carb intake.

Like I mentioned previously, ketones lead to more balanced neurotransmitters, particularly between GABA and glutamate. While glutamate is responsible for promoting stimulation, GABA is the one that takes care of reducing stimulation in the body. More often than not, lack of focus and brain fog are caused by very low GABA and way too much glutamate. This usually happens when the brain uses glutamic acid and glutamate for energy. Ketone bodies can restore the balance between these important neurotransmitters.

When there is a balance between GABA and glutamate, you can have a much better focus. You will feel a better sense of calmness. And you will feel less anxious and stressed out.

You become more energized.

The ketogenic diet paves the way to better mitochondrial function. At the same time, it produces fewer reactive oxygen species. But what does this have to do with energy?

An improved mitochondrial function happens to lead to more energy for the cells. With fewer reactive oxygen species, you also get to improve and promote energy efficiency. This means that keto helps you maximize your cells and realize full energy potential.

You get to avoid inflammation and reduce pain.

When there are less reactive oxygen species, the body does not have to keep repairing damage as frequently. Lesser damage means reduced inflammation levels. And if you are suffering from chronic pain, your pain will be reduced as well.

Chapter 5 – Best Ways of Achieving Ketosis

You now understand the importance of ketosis and how much you can benefit from it but how much do you really want it? Let's get real. Entering ketosis is not a piece of cake. It takes time and a lot of sacrifices. It requires planning. Unfortunately, you can't simply cut off your carbs and cross your fingers until you get to that state. But if you're ready for the challenge, please put your game face on and get ready to work!

There are various ways to enter a state of ketosis. The following methods have been proven by science to help you achieve ketosis quicker.

Minimize Your Carb Intake.

Cutting most of your carbs may not be enough to get your body into ketosis but it's an important factor and probably the most essential one. We've gone through how the body cells make use of glucose as the main source of energy earlier. With a very low carb intake, the cells will become resourceful enough to find alternative fuel sources. Such alternative sources include fatty acids and ketone bodies.

The body likes to save up so extra glucose gets stored in the muscles and the liver to form glycogen. When you significantly reduce your carb consumption, stored glycogen gets used and insulin levels decline. This step is very important because it paves the way for the release of fatty acids from the fat storage in your body.

As fatty acids are released, the liver gets creative and converts them into ketone bodies in the form of acetone, acetoacetate, and beta-hydroxybutyrate. As you've learned earlier, some of the ketones are also used as brain fuel. Now the question is, how low is very low carb?

Here's the tricky part. Some people may be considered biologically lucky because they will find it much easier to enter ketosis. On the other hand, some will find it challenging indeed. It will take more time and greater restriction. So while some people will do just fine taking 40 grams of carbs a day, there are others who may need to reduce theirs to as low as 20 grams a day or even lower.

Aside from the biological factor, you also need to consider your main objective for wanting to achieve ketosis. Are you aiming to lose weight? Or are you trying to use it as a therapeutic diet?

If your goal is to lose weight and get into a fitter shape or to bring your blood sugar to a healthier level or to reduce your risk to heart diseases, targeting a blood ketone level between 0.5–3.0 mmol/L may be the suitable strategy. In this case, carb consumption should be limited to 20 to 50 grams a day.

If you have a specific health condition you want to address, you can go into a therapeutic ketogenic diet. This is especially recommended for people suffering from epilepsy or as part of an alternative cancer therapy. It is much more restrictive at 15 grams of carbs a day or less. Let me emphasize however, that to effectively and safely use keto for therapeutic purposes, you should do it under professional supervision.

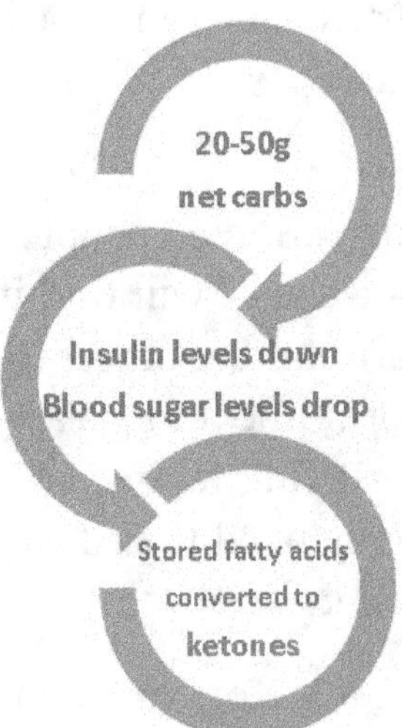

For the majority, keeping your carb intake between 20 and 50 grams of net carbs a day is enough to reduce insulin and blood sugar levels that will eventually lead to stored fatty acid release for the liver to convert into ketones.

Try Intermittent Fasting.

Fasting is another way for you to achieve ketosis. I know a lot of people are quite skeptical about fasting because the idea of starving themselves is repulsive. Don't panic just yet.

Did you know that a lot of people actually enter ketosis between dinner time and breakfast? You could be one of those people too! Sure, it is a mild ketosis but it demonstrates how natural fasting really is to all of us. Unless you sneak out to the fridge in the middle of the night, you're fasting until you break that fast.

Intermittent fasting is simply a dietary approach that usually involves short-term but regular fasts which can help in inducing ketosis. Let's say you usually break your fast in the morning at 7 am. Intermittent fasting simply suggests that you postpone the meal and take it at 11 am or at noon. The idea is to give yourself 16 hours without food and limiting your meals to an 8-hour window. Essentially, you are encouraged to skip breakfast but you can still have coffee, of course, tea or water as long as you make sure to keep the sugar out.

If you like kingly breakfast so much that you can't let it go, here's another option for you. What about a fat fasting? In this approach, you are encouraged to limit your daily calorie intake to 1,000 with 85 to about 90 percent of that calorie portion from fat. It is another possible way for you to achieve the state of ketosis more quickly.

If you're taking the fat fast route, do so for no longer than 3 to 5 days. With a low calorie and low protein consumption, excessive fat fasting can lead to excessive muscle loss. A max of 3 to 5 days will keep you on the safe side.

Make Sure to Get Enough Protein but Not Too Much.

Adequate but not excessive protein intake is helpful in making your body enter ketosis. In some cases, lower than adequate protein may be necessary to maximize ketone levels such as in the case of cancer and epilepsy patients. Keep in mind, however, that these patients' diets are medically supervised. For the general population, restricting protein intake to very low amounts for the sake of increasing ketone production isn't healthy at all. Let's remind ourselves why protein is important.

First reason goes to gluconeogenesis. For this process to happen, the liver needs an adequate supply of amino acids which comes from protein. Why is gluconeogenesis important? Aren't we focusing on ketosis?

Although most of the human body can survive and function just fine using ketones as fuel, there are some cells and organs that can't use them. This group includes portions of the brain, some parts of the kidneys and red blood cells. Gluconeogenesis makes sure that these parts of the body don't get left behind. And so in this process, the very reliable liver makes new glucose from amino acids which it supplies exclusively to these ketone snobs.

The second reason goes to muscle mass. If you fast too much or don't get enough protein from your diet, you put yourself at risk of losing muscle mass. If you intend to maintain that mass, you should maintain an adequate protein consumption. While it is a given that fat loss typically goes hand in hand with muscle loss in the process of losing weight, it's also important to preserve some mass and you can do this by making sure you still get enough protein while restricting your carb intake.

According to studies, you can maximize your physical performance and preserve muscle mass if you keep your protein consumption within the range of 1.2–1.7 grams per kilogram or 0.55–0.77 grams per pound of lean mass (Phinney, 2004). Weight loss studies agree to this range. Researchers found that restricting carbs while maintaining moderate protein intake helps in inducing and maintaining a state of ketosis. As a matter of fact, one study found that staying on a ketogenic diet with 30 percent of the calories coming from protein and keeping at it for 4 weeks resulted to an average of 1.52 mmol/L blood ketone level in 17 obese men. This level is within the nutritional ketosis range of 0.5–3.0 mmol/L (Johnstone et al, 2008).

With all these said, it can still be confusing for you figuring out how much is enough and how much is considered excessive. Let's use your digits. To compute your protein requirements on a keto diet, you can use the following formula.

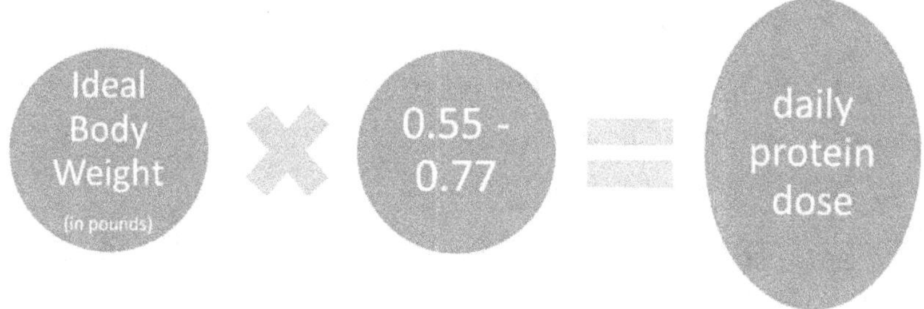

So let's say, your current weight is 180 pounds or 82 kilograms but your goal is to be at 130 pounds or 59 kilograms. Using the formula above, your recommended protein intake on a ketogenic diet is between 71 and 100 grams per day. Going below this range will likely cause you loss of muscle mass but going above it will inhibit ketone production. Best to stay within the recommended range.

Get More Fat from High Quality, Healthy Sources.

To boost ketone levels and reach ketosis, you will need to increase your consumption of healthy fat. This is why the ketogenic diet is designed to be high in fat, moderate in protein and very low in carbs. Your typical keto diet consists of 60 to about 80 percent fat. In fact, the keto diet for epilepsy patients contains even higher at 85 to 90 percent.

It's not all about amplifying fat, however. Rather it is very important to choose healthy fat sources. So don't worry, you don't have to down a bottle of cooking oil. Fat can be excellent for you as long as it is from high-quality sources.

What exactly are healthy fats? Healthy fats include avocado, olive oil, coconut oil, lard, butter and tallow among others.

Healthy fat can come from both animal and plant sources. We'll get into this a little bit further in the next chapters.

Give Coconut Oil a Shot.

Coconut oil should be on your list of healthy fats. It's healthy and it can help your body through ketosis more quickly. What's so special about coconut oil anyway?

I've mentioned medium-chain triglycerides or MCTs in the previous chapter. Coconut oil contains MCTs which makes it very special indeed. Compared to other fats, MCTs are taken directly and absorbed more rapidly into the liver so they can be immediately used for fuel or converted into ketone bodies. Studies found that coconut oil is actually among the best ways to elevate ketone levels in Alzheimer's patients and people suffering from other nervous system disorders (Fernando et al, 2015).

There are a total of four types of MCTs found in coconut oil. A bulk of it, around 50 percent is from lauric acid. Research suggests that sources of fat with greater lauric acid percentage can possibly lead to a better-sustained ketosis. The main reason for this is that lauric acid compared to other types of MCTs tend to become metabolized in a more gradual manner (Nonaka, 2016).

Before you get into downing some coconut oil, please bear in mind that adding it slowly significantly helps in minimizing digestive side effects such as diarrhea or stomach cramping. The safest way is to start with just one teaspoon a day. You can gradually increase your intake to 2 or up to 3 tablespoons a day in a week.

Increase Your Physical Activity.

Ketosis is not only beneficial for people who want to lose weight or prevent and possibly treat health conditions. More studies reveal that being in this metabolic state may also benefit athletic performance particularly endurance exercise (Cox & Clarke, 2014). At the same time, ramping up your physical activity level can also help you achieve ketosis.

Through exercise, you can burn your glycogen storage. On a normal diet with high carbs, glycogen storage will become replenished. However, as you restrict your carb consumption, you can manage to keep your glycogen storage down. The liver responds by increasing ketone production. Your muscles can then rely on ketones as the new fuel source.

In one study, researchers found that exercise effectively increased the production rate of ketones in individuals with low blood ketone levels. On the other hand, exercise can possibly decrease blood ketone levels for a short period of time among those with already high blood ketone concentrations (Féry & Balasse, 1986).

A small study published in the Medicine and Science in Sports and Exercise, found just how much of an effect physical activity has on ketosis. The blood ketone levels of 9 older women were tested. The researchers found that the subjects' blood ketone rose to about 137 up to 314 percent higher when they engaged in a physical activity before a meal. Their results were higher than when exercise was scheduled after a meal (Borek et al, 2009).

If your body finds it challenging to get into ketosis, you can ramp up your level of physical activity to help you get there. Keep in mind, however, that it will probably take roughly 1 to 4 weeks before your body properly adapts to using fatty acids and ketones as its primary source of energy. So while you're giving your body some time to adjust to these changes, you may feel a slight reduction in your physical performance although this will only occur temporarily (Phinney, 2004).

Monitor Your Ketone Levels and Make Adjustments to Your Diet Accordingly.

Entering and maintaining ketosis is not the same for everyone. I've laid out a couple of suggestions earlier in this chapter about diet composition. But to make sure you're on the right track, I would strongly recommend that you test your ketone levels. This is important so you can find out if you are within your goals. Otherwise, you can make the necessary adjustments in your diet in line with your personal objectives. So how do you test for ketones?

First of all, you should understand that there are 3 types of ketones. These are the following:

- acetone
- beta-hydroxybutyrate
- acetoacetate

Traces of these ketones are usually found in the blood, urine and in your breath.

1. Measuring ketone levels through your breath.

Acetone, specifically, can be found in the breath. A couple of studies confirm that measuring acetone breath levels is indeed a reliable method of monitoring ketosis for individuals following a ketogenic diet (Musa-Veloso, Likhodii, & Cunnane, 2002). One way of doing this is through the Ketonix meter. It specifically measures acetone level in the breath. All you need to do is breathe into it. A color will then flash indicating whether or not you're in ketosis and the level you're at.

2. Measuring ketone levels through your blood.

The ketone beta-hydroxybutyrate can be traced through the blood. The accuracy of measuring the BHB amount in the blood has been confirmed by studies to be a reliable indicator of ketosis level (Wallace, Meston, Gardner, & Matthews, 2001).

A blood ketone meter works like a glucose meter. All you need is a tiny blood drop which should be placed on a strip. You will then insert the strip into the ketone meter. This can be an expensive option because the strips, in particular, are a little costly.

3. Measuring ketone levels through urine.

The final item on our list, acetoacetate, can be measured in urine. In this process, ketone urine strips are to be dipped into your urine. The color of the strip will turn into various shades of purple or pink. The color it gives out shall indicate your level of ketosis. As a general rule, darker colored strips indicate a higher level of ketones.

Compared to a blood ketone meter, ketone urine strips tend to be much easier to use and also inexpensive. The major downside is that the accuracy of results is not as well defined. However, this will probably work out just fine if you just need to confirm that you've stepped into a ketosis state.

All three methods seem to work and you can choose any of them to measure and monitor your ketosis level. This way, you know exactly where you stand.

Follow the Ketogenic Diet.

The best route to ketosis is probably the ketogenic diet. The diet offers the healthiest and safest way for you to reap the benefit of ketosis. By limiting carbs but maintaining enough caloric consumption mainly from fat and protein, the diet allows the body to go through the ketogenic process while preserving muscle tissue. Through ketosis and by using ketone bodies, you create fuel without the need to burn off your precious muscle mass.

The diet actually comes in many forms.

1. Standard Ketogenic Diet - It consists of high fat, moderate protein, and a very low carb. It usually recommends 75 percent fat, 20 percent protein and the remaining 5 percent to carbs.

2. Cyclical Ketogenic Diet - This version involves certain periods of high carb refeeds. For instance, on a weekly schedule, 5 days is dedicated to following the standard ketogenic diet and the remaining 2 becomes high-carb days.

3. Targeted Ketogenic Diet - In this version of the diet, you are allowed to include more carbs to supplement your workouts.

4. High-protein Ketogenic Diet - This version is somewhat similar to the standard but a little bit more of protein is added, taking some percent from the fat portion. The diet will consist of 60 percent fat, 35 percent protein and only 5 percent carbs.

Targeted and Cyclical ketogenic diets are recommended for athletes and bodybuilders since they are more advanced versions of the diet. The ones that have been researched on extensively are the High-protein and Standard ketogenic diets. Since you're a newbie to this, the standard version is most advisable. As such, it will be our focus in this book.

Chapter 6 - Foods that Will Slow Ketosis Down

Basically, this is how your daily portions should look like. Since getting the exact percentages right is almost impossible, I'm giving you a range here: 70-80% fat, 20-25% protein and let's keep carbs limited to 5% or lower. As long as you keep within the range, you'll be fine.

From this pie itself, you already know that high carb foods are a big no-no. If you go above the range with either protein or carb-centric foods, you can quickly be brought out of ketosis. This will further slow the process down and impede your body's ability to burn fat.

So in this chapter, I'm bringing you a list of foods to absolutely avoid on a keto diet. To make it even easier, I'm grouping them according to macronutrient. That's right, high carbs are not the only one on the restricted list. There are certain protein and fat foods that you should definitely avoid to. Let's get on with it.

A Big NO for these Carbs

1. Grains

We don't negotiate when it comes to grains. ALL grains are off limits. And yes, even whole grains should not be considered. Refer to the chart below to understand why.

	CARB CONTENT	PROTEIN CONTENT	FAT CONTENT
AMARANTH	46g	9g	4g
BARLEY	44g	4g	1g
BULGUR	33g	5.6g	0.4g
BUCKWHEAT	33g	6g	1g
CORN	32g	4g	1g
MILLET	41g	6g	2g
OATS	26g	6g	3g
QUINOA	39g	8g	4g
RICE	45g	5g	2g
RYE (per slice of bread)	15g	3g	1g
SORGHUM	39g	5g	1g
SPROUTED GRAINS (per slice of bread)	15g	4g	0.5g
WHEAT (per slice of bread)	14g	3g	1g

NOTE: Measurements are based on 1 cup of cooked grains unless otherwise stated.

It goes without saying that all bread, pastas, crackers, pizza crusts and cookies made from any of these grains are prohibited.

2. Beans and Legumes

These are indeed good to have on a regular diet. However, they have no place in a keto diet mainly because they have a very high starch content.

	CARB CONTENT	PROTEIN CONTENT	FAT CONTENT
BLACK BEANS	23g	7g	0.5g
BLACK EYED PEAS	14g	2g	0g
CANNELLINI BEANS	18g	6g	0.5g
CHICKPEAS	20g	6g	2g
FAVA BEANS	17g	6g	0g
GREAT NORTHERN BEANS	22g	8g	0g
GREEN PEAS	14g	4g	0g
KIDNEY BEANS	18.5g	7g	0.75g
LENTILS	19g	8g	0g
LIMA BEANS	19g	6g	0g
PINTO BEANS	20g	7g	0g

NOTE: Macro calculations are based on 1/2 cup of cooked beans and legumes.

3. Most Fruits

Yes, fruits are healthy indeed but in order to be compliant with keto, it is best to avoid them. Why does keto ban fruits when they are good for you? It is simply because most of them have a very high carb and sugar content. The list includes dried fruits, fruit juices, tropical fruits and fruit smoothies.

If you must eat some, you better choose the lower-sugar ones such as raspberries, blackberries, and blueberries. And even if these fruit options are lower in sugar and carbs, please don't go crazy about eating them. Remember, you only have 5 percent allowance for carbs. Eat them sparingly.

	CARB CONTENT	PROTEIN CONTENT	FAT CONTENT
APPLE (1 medium)	22g	0g	0g
BANANA (1 small)	18.5g	0.9g	0.2g
GRAPES (1 cup)	27g	1g	0g
MANGO (1 medium)	50g	3g	1g
ORANGE (1 medium)	17g	1g	0.3g
PAPAYA (1 small)	15g	0.9g	0.2g
PINEAPPLE (1/2 cup)	18g	1g	0g
TANGERINE (1 medium)	12g	1g	0g
DRIED FRUITS (1 cup of raisins/ dried mango/ dates, etc.)	57g	2g	0g
FRUIT CONCENTRATE (2 fl.oz. of apple juice concentrate)	29g	0g	0g
FRUIT JUICE (1 cup of orange juice)	26g	2g	0g
FRUIT SYRUP (2 tbsp of blueberry syrup)	15g	0g	0g

4. Starchy Vegetables

Vegetables are healthy but a lot of them also contain too much starch. High starch is equivalent to high carbs and eating them will defeat the purpose of keto. As a general rule, stay away from those that grow beneath the ground. When it comes to vegetables on keto, leafy greens are your best friend!

	CARB CONTENT	PROTEIN CONTENT	FAT CONTENT
CARROTS	6g	1g	0g
CORN	32g	4g	1g
CHERRY TOMATOES (1 cup raw)	6g	1.3g	0.3g
PARSNIPS	15g	1g	0.3g
PEAS	14g	4g	0g
POTATOES (1 medium baked)	28g	3g	0.3g
SWEET POTATOES	14g	1g	0g
YAMS	19g	1g	0g
YUCCA (1 cup raw)	39g	1.5g	0g

NOTE: Macro calculations are based on 1/2 cup of vegetables unless otherwise stated.

5. SUGAR

Sugar can come under many different names on labels and under the guise of different forms. Some may seem like a better option. However, in keto, sugar is sugar.

	CARB CONTENT	PROTEIN CONTENT	FAT CONTENT
AGAVE NECTAR	14g	0g	0g
CANE SUGAR	12g	0g	0g
HIGH-FRUCTOSE CORN SYRUP	14g	0g	0g
HONEY	17g	0g	0g
MAPLE SYRUP	14g	0g	0g
RAW SUGAR	12g	0g	0g
TURBINADO SUGAR	12g	0g	0g

NOTE: Macro calculations are based on 1 tablespoon of sugar.

If you love dessert, don't worry about it. There are keto dessert options that you can enjoy too.

Won't I need more carbs because of my active lifestyle?

If you are an active person who is used to carbo loading after working out, you may wonder if you're an exception. Unless you are a competitive athlete or a bodybuilder, sorry to burst your bubble but there's no getting around the carb restriction. Yes, it applies to you, average person working on building muscles, you don't have to worry yourself about getting extra carb or protein. You may increase your overall daily calories but you should still follow the keto macronutrient ratio (70-80% fat, 20-25% protein, and <5% carbs).

STAY AWAY from these Protein Sources

Surprised? You may think all protein is okay but they aren't. And you'll find out why.

1. Milk and Low-Fat Dairy

There's nothing wrong with raw milk as long as you take them in small amounts and keep within your daily carb allowance. Full-fat dairy products such as sour cream, heavy cream, butter, and yogurt are also alright. All other types of milk including the reduced- and low-fat dairy product options are to be avoided at all cost. That's because they contain too many carbs. Also, pasteurized milk is quite challenging for some people to digest. They lack beneficial bacteria and most have harmful hormones content.

	CARB CONTENT	PROTEIN CONTENT	FAT CONTENT
MILK (1 cup of 2% milk)	12g	8g	5g
SHREDDED CHEESE (1/2 cup)	2g	14g	18g
EVAPORATED SKIM MILK (1 cup)	14g	10g	0.2g
FAT-FREE BUTTER SUBSTITUTES (1 tbsp)	0.63g	0g	0.4g
FAT-FREE or LOW-FAT YOGURT (1 container)	16g	0g	0g
LOW-FAT CREAM CHEESE (1 tbsp)	1g	2g	2.6g
LOW-FAT WHIPPED TOPPING (2 tbsp)	16g	0g	0g

2. Factory Farmed Animal Products

As much as possible, you should go for the grass-fed and organic animal products. Grain-fed meats and dairy products are to be avoided because they are usually lower in nutritional content. Factory-farmed pork and fish should also be banned from your diet because they contain too much omega-6 which is inflammatory when taken in large amounts. Also, factory-farmed fish often have high mercury content.

You should also stay away from processed meats such as packaged sausages and hot dogs. Most if not all of them contain nitrates. These substances are downright harmful and can possibly increase your risk of cancer.

3. Soy Products

Because they are low carb, soy products seem to fit right with keto. However, there are a couple of issues with them. One, they contain high levels of phytoestrogens and such can have negative effects on your hormone levels. Two, most of them are highly processed. And this means they are likely to contain phytoestrogens in concentrated amounts while giving you much fewer nutrients. Three, they are rich in phytates which tend to cause the binding of minerals that will lead to absorption issues.

Soy products including soy milk, tofu and soy-based meat substitutes and dairy can inhibit ketosis and are best avoided. There are a few exceptions, however. One of which is the soy sauce alternative, fermented soy. For instance, you'll do just fine with a tamari sauce that is gluten-free.

WATCH OUT for These Fat Foods

Let me emphasize again that there are two kinds of fat, the good one, and the bad kind. Nutritious, unprocessed oils like macadamia nut oils, virgin olive oil, and coconut oil are the kind you want to get loads of. They are excellent sources of both unsaturated and saturated fat. What you need to avoid are the unhealthy oils including the following vegetable oils.

CANOLA OIL	SAFFLOWER OIL
CORN OIL	SESAME OIL
GRAPESEED OIL	SOYBEAN OIL
PEANUT OIL	SUNFLOWER OIL

What to Drink on a Ketogenic Diet?

Water is the best drink you can have on a ketogenic diet. Drinking calories on keto and any kind of diet for that matter is best avoided. But there are drinks you can't afford to indulge in unless you want to jeopardize your ketosis.

1. Alcohol

One of the easiest and quickest way to impede the keto process is to drink alcoholic beverages. They are also high in carbs.

	CARB CONTENT	PROTEIN CONTENT	FAT CONTENT
BEERS (12 fl.oz.)	12.7g	1.6g	0g
COCKTAILS (1 cocktail)	5g	0.1g	0g
FLAVORED LIQUORS (1 fl.oz.)	3-6g	0g	0g
MIXERS with juices, flavored syrups, and sodas (2 Fl.oz. of Margarita Mixer)	12g	0g	0g
WINES (1 glass of sweet wine)	14g	0.2g	0g

If you must drink, choose hard liquor instead. Although hard liquor is from carb sources too, the sugars in them are converted into ethyl alcohol in the process of distillation and fermentation. Alcohol is ethanol. That means it's readily available to be converted into sugar. From the perspective of the cell, a glass of wine is no different from a can of soda.

2. Sweetened Beverages

Sugary drinks should be among the items at the top of the things to avoid on a ketogenic diet. They will destroy you. The list includes sweetened milk products as well as coffee and tea with added sweeteners. Without the sweeteners, brewed coffee and tea are fine choices.

	CARB CONTENT	PROTEIN CONTENT	FAT CONTENT
All Sugar-Sweetened Sodas (1 can)	36g	0.2g	0g
Bottled or Fresh Fruit/ Vegetable Juices (1 cup)	18g	0.1g	0g
Bottled or Fresh Fruit/ Vegetable Smoothies (1 cup)	34g	0.8g	0.2g

All diet sodas are prohibited. They all contain artificial sweeteners which disrupt blood sugar levels and jeopardizes ketosis. They lack nutritional value and they increase cravings. Even if you're not on keto, they're just bad for you.

OTHER Keto Devils to Avoid

1. Processed and Packaged Foods

Packaged products are filled with trans fats, extra sugar, preservatives and other junk you can think of. Almond milk and other products containing carrageenan, gelatin, dried fruits and others containing sulfites as well as all sodas and soft drinks should be avoided. If you look at the following list, you may see minimal carb content but these food items are bad for you because of all the junk they contain.

	CARB CONTENT	PROTEIN CONTENT	FAT CONTENT
CANDIES (1 piece)	9g	0g	0g
Commercially baked goods such as cakes and cookies (1 piece of cookie)	30g	2g	10g
ICE CREAM (1 cup)	2g	4.7g	14.2g
MARGARINES (1 tbsp)	0.63g	0g	0.4g
WHEAT GLUTEN (1/2 cup)	2g	46g	1g

You should especially watch out for packaged foods that are marketed as "zero-carb" or "low-carb." Although they may indeed be low in carbohydrates per serving, they are often too tiny. You won't be satisfied with just one. These tiny little devils will make you want more and the next thing you know you're way off ketosis. They also usually contain artificial flavors and additives and probably gluten too. If you want to reach and stay in ketosis, you should stick to whole foods.

2. Artificial Sweeteners

You will probably find mixed information about artificial sweeteners. They should be treated with caution as they may affect your blood sugar levels. They may also cause craving issues. There are some people whose ketosis may be disrupted as a result of these sweeteners.

Stay cautious about these Artificial Sweeteners	
ACESULFAME	SACCHARIN
ASPARTAME	SPLENDA
EQUAL	SUCRALOSE

3. Condiments

I suggest that you make your own condiments. Use pure herbs and spices. If you can't however, just make sure to stay away from those made with unhealthy oils and added sugars. And never be fooled by those labeled as "low-fat."

Chapter 7 - KETO-Friendly Foods

Seeing the long list of what not to eat from the previous chapter may seem like you're left with nothing but water. Don't fret. You actually have great options. This chapter will point you in the direction of nutritious foods that will absolutely help you to ketosis and stay there for the long run. Let's get on with the most keto-friendly foods you can chow down on!

Fats and Oils

Incredibly satiating and delicious, fats are essential in keeping at ketosis. The key here is to choose the right kind. A good balance between omega 3 and omega-6 fatty acids is essential for promoting overall health. So here's to give you an idea.

	FAT CONTENT	PROTEIN CONTENT	NET CARB CONTENT
BUTTER or GHEE (1 tbsp)	11.5g	0.12g	0g
COCONUT BUTTER (1 tbsp)	10.5g	1g	1.5g
COCONUT OIL (1 tbsp)	13.47g	0g	0g
DRIPPING/ LARD (1 tbsp)	12.8g	0g	0g
FLAXSEED OIL (1 tbsp)	13.6g	0g	0g
MAYONNAISE (1 tbsp)	10.33g	0.13g	0.08g
MCT POWDER (1 scoop)	7g	0.5g	0g
MCT OIL (1 tbsp)	14g	0g	0g
OLIVE OIL (1 tbsp)	13.5g	0g	0g
SESAME SEED OIL (1 tbsp)	13.6g	0g	0g
WALNUT OIL (1 tbsp)	13.6g	0g	0g

Nuts and seeds are also a great source of fat. However, they also contain some amount of carbs particularly almonds, pistachios, and cashews. Eat them sparingly.

NUTS AND SEEDS	FAT CONTENT	PROTEIN CONTENT	NET CARB CONTENT
ALMOND BUTTER no salt (1 tbsp)	9g	3.5g	1.5g
ALMONDS (23 pcs)	14g	6g	2.5g
ALMOND FLOUR/ MEAL (1/4 cup)	11g	6g	3g
NUTS AND SEEDS	FAT CONTENT	PROTEIN CONTENT	NET CARB CONTENT
BRAZIL NUTS (5 pcs)	17g	3.5g	1g
CASHEW (1/4 cup)	12g	4g	9g
CASHEW BUTTER (1 tbsp)	8g	3g	4g
COCONUT unsweetened, shredded (1/4 cup)	7g	1g	1g
HAZELNUTS (12 pcs)	10g	2.5g	1.5g
MACADAMIAS (6 kernels)	11g	1g	0.8g
MACADAMIA BUTTER (1 tbsp)	10g	2g	1g
PECANS (10 halves)	10g	1.3g	0. 5g
PEANUT BUTTER chunky salted (1 tbsp)	8g	4g	2g
PEANUT BUTTER smooth salted (1 tbsp)	8g	3.5g	3g

PILI NUTS (1/4 cup)	**24g**	**3g**	**0g**
PINE NUTS (2 tbsp)	**14g**	**2.7g**	**0.7g**
PISTACHIOS (25 pcs)	**8g**	**3.5g**	**3g**
PUMPKIN SEEDS hulled (2 tbsp)	**14g**	**9g**	**1g**
SESAME SEEDS (2 tbsp)	**9g**	**3.2g**	**2g**
SUNFLOWER SEEDS hulled (1/4 cup)	**15g**	**6g**	**3g**
SUNFLOWER SEED BUTTER (1 tbsp)	**9g**	**2.8g**	**3g**
TAHINI sesame paste (1 tbsp)	**8g**	**2.6g**	**2g**
WALNUTS (7 halves)	**9g**	**2g**	**1g**

Low-Carb Vegetables

When it comes to vegetables on the ketogenic diet, you should only remember this: no to root vegetables and yes to leafy greens. The magic in dark leafy greens is that they are rich in nutrients and low in carbs which make them absolutely perfect for keto. If you stay with kale and spinach or anything that resembles them, you'll be alright.

What if you're not the biggest fan of leafy greens? Do you have any other choice? Of course, you do! Choose vegetables that are grown above ground. Those from the cruciferous family are best.

You can do more than just make a salad out of vegetables. You can roast them or sauté them. The options are endless. You just have to put your creativity hat on.

Below you will find a list of keto-friendly vegetables along with their carbs and fiber content.

	TOTAL CARB CONTENT	FIBER CONTENT	NET CARBS
ARTICHOKE HEARTS	2.97g	1.6g	1.37g
ARUGULA	3.65g	1.6g	2.05g
ASPARAGUS	3.88g	2.1g	1.78g
AVOCADO	8.64g	6.8g	1.84g
BAMBOO SHOOTS	5.2g	2.2g	3g
BEAN SPROUTS	5.94g	1.8g	4.14g
BELL PEPPER	4.6g	1.7g	2.9g
BOK CHOI	2.18g	1g	1.18g
BROCCOLI	6.64g	2.6g	4.04g
BROCCOLI RAAB	2.85g	2.7g	0.15g
BRUSSELS SPROUTS	8.95g	3.8g	5.15g
CABBAGE (green)	6.1g	3.1g	3g
CABBAGE (red)	7.37g	2.1g	5.27g
CABBAGE (white)	5.37g	2.3g	3.07g
CARROTS	9.58g	2.8g	6.78g
CAULIFLOWER	4.97g	2g	2.97g
CELERIAC	9.2g	1.8g	7.4g
CELERY	2.97g	1.6g	1.37g
CUCUMBER	3.63g	0.5g	3.13g
EGGPLANT	5.88g	3g	2.88g
FENNEL	7.3g	3.1g	4.2g
GINGER	17.77g	2g	15.77g
GREEN BEANS	6.97g	2.7g	4.27g
JALAPENO PEPPER	6.5g	2.8g	3.7g
KALE	8.75g	3.6g	5.15g
KOHLRABI	6.2g	3.6g	2.6g
LEEK	14.15g	1.8g	12.35

VEGETABLES	TOTAL CARB CONTENT	FIBER CONTENT	NET CARBS
MUSHROOMS	3.26g	1g	2.26g
MUSTARD GREENS	4.67g	3.2g	1.47g
NOPALES	3.33g	2.2g	1.13g
OKRA	7.45g	3.2g	4.25g
OLIVES	6g	3.2g	2.8g
ONION	9.34g	1.7g	7.64g
PUMPKIN	7g	1g	6g
RADISH	3.4g	1.6g	1.8g
RUTABAGA	8.62g	2.3g	6.32g
SNOW PEAS	7.55g	2.6g	4.95g
SPINACH	3.63g	2.2g	1.43g
SWISS CHARD	3.74g	1.6g	2.14g
TOMATO	3.89g	1.2g	2.69g
TURNIPS	6.43g	1.6g	4.83g
WATERCRESS	1.29g	0.5g	0.79g
ZUCCHINI	3.11g	1g	2.11g

Note: Macro calculations are based on 100g of vegetables

From the list of low carb vegetables above, the following come highly recommended. They are very rich in micronutrients and are also low in net carbs. You have to make sure to get them on your plate.

1. Broccoli

Touted as a superfood, broccoli is super in its vitamin C and K content. There are studies that have found that this vegetable can actually help in decreasing insulin resistance especially in people with type 2 diabetes. They are also great anti-cancer veggies. All these nutrients will only cost you 4g of net carbs per cup.

2. Asparagus

This green is more than just a great side dish. You can have it with bacon wrapped around and enjoy with aioli. You can chop it for stir-fries or grill it.

Asparagus is especially rich in vitamins A, C, and K. It may help in reducing anxiety levels. At the same time, it can promote brain health.

3. Mushrooms

Mushrooms can bring an otherwise boring dish to life by adding flavor to it. At only 1g net carb a cup, mushrooms possess anti-inflammatory properties.

4. Zucchini

This great noodle replacement boasts of a meager 3g net carbs a cup. It is also a great vitamin C source.

5. Spinach

A cup of cooked spinach only gives you 3g of net carbs which makes it an excellent way of bulking up your keto lunch with a salad. According to studies, spinach helps in reducing your risk to common eye diseases. It also promotes heart health as this leafy green is packed with vitamins and minerals.

6. Avocado

Technically, avocado is a fruit but they are usually used as an alternative to a lot of vegetables. And they are a perfect keto food because they supplement your fat intake. High in monounsaturated fats, avocados help in reducing LDL or bad cholesterol and triglycerides. They are also packed with potassium and vitamin C which aids in relieving electrolyte issues.

7. Cauliflower

A great alternative for mashed potatoes, casseroles, pizza and wraps, cauliflower is truly a versatile vegetable. With only 2g of net carbs a cup, cauliflower is among the most commonly used veggies in a keto diet. It is also rich in vitamins C and K. This vegetable is hailed for its ability to help fight heart diseases and cancer.

8. Bell Peppers

These colorful ones are very nutritious. They are high in vitamin A. Bell peppers also possess anti-inflammatory properties.

9. Green Beans

Most legumes are too high in carbs but green beans are an exception. Also known as snap beans, green beans help in the improvement of brain function. A cup of these only costs you 6g of net carbs.

10. Lettuce and Kale

What will a salad be without lettuce or kale? Both are very nutritious and boasts of their vitamins A and C content. They help in reducing your risk of heart diseases. Kale is a little bit ahead of lettuce when it comes to nutritional content but it is also a little higher on the carb scale. So when you do have some kale, make sure you are still within your daily carb allowance.

Bone Broth

In addition to the vegetables mentioned earlier, bone broth is another keto-friendly food you would want to have in your weekly menu. It is regarded as a healing superfood. It is rich in minerals and amino acids.

Cutting out processed foods from your diet can cause an electrolyte imbalance. Bone broth can save the day and restore the balance. It also helps in detoxification and eases one of the side effects of ketosis which is keto flu.

Bone broth can be prepared using animal bones from venison, lamb, beef, turkey, chicken or fish. You get the best out of them by boiling them in a crock pot for 24 to 48 hours.

Dairy Products

Most dairies make it to the keto door. The key to dairy is to choose the full-fat version. Raw and organic are also ideal. Always opt for dairy with high-quality fat. Here are a few to load up on.

	FAT CONTENT	PROTEIN CONTENT	NET CARB CONTENT
BLUE CHEESE (1 oz.)	8g	6g	0. 7g
BRIE (1 oz.)	8g	6g	0.1g
CHEDDAR or COLBY (1 oz.)	9.5g	6.5g	1g
COTTAGE CHEESE creamed (1/2 cup)	4.5g	11.7g	3.5g
COTTAGE CHEESE 2% fat (1/2 cup)	2.5g	12g	5g
CREAM CHEESE (2 tbsp)	10g	2g	0.6g
FETA (1 oz.)	6g	4g	1g
GOAT CHEESE soft (1 oz.)	6g	5g	0g

GOUDA (1 oz.)	**8g**	**7g**	**0.6g**
HEAVY WHIPPING CREAM or DOUBLE CREAM fluid (1 tbsp)	**5.4g**	**0.4g**	**0.4g**
HEAVY WHIPPING CREAM or DOUBLE CREAM whipped (1/2 cup)	**22g**	**1.7g**	**1.6g**
MOZZARELLA whole milk (1 oz.)	**6.3g**	**6.3g**	**0.6g**
PARMESAN (1 oz.)	**7.3g**	**10g**	**1g**
RICOTTA whole milk (1/2 cup)	**16g**	**14g**	**4g**
SOUR CREAM (1 tbsp)	**2.3g**	**0.3g**	**0.6g**
SWISS (1 oz.)	**9g**	**7.6g**	**0.4g**
YOGURT plain unsweetened, whole milk (4 oz.)	**3.7g**	**4g**	**5.3g**

Fatty Cuts of Meat

Fatty cuts allow you to level up on your keto fat intake. They are also incredibly tasty. You may be used to lean cuts but it's time to double down on fat. So don't be afraid to go for your favorite succulent cut.

Fish and Seafood

A quality source of protein, fish, and seafood are also rich in omega-3 fatty acids!

The best fishes with loads of omega-3 include salmon, tuna, mackerel, halibut, trout, cod, mahi-mahi, and catfish among others. As for selfish, your best bets are lobster, mussels, crab, clams, and oysters.

Meat and Poultry

Meat from goat, lamb, beef, and pork give you much-needed protein with keto-friendly fat. If you like pork, you'd be happy to indulge yourself in pork loin, chops, and tenderloin. Ham and bacon are also good as long as they are not the processed and packaged kind. And when it comes to beef, the fattier cuts are preferable including steak, roast, ground beef, veal, and stews.

Poultry is also among the most preferable for ketosis because of the dark fatty meats. Chicken, duck, turkey, quail and wild game are recommended. As for eggs, you should use whole ones. They can be boiled, scrambled, fried or deviled.

Low-Carb Fruits

Most fruits can ruin ketosis because they are rich in sugar. With the exception of avocados, you can enjoy the ones on this list in very small amounts.

	TOTAL CARB CONTENT	FIBER CONTENT	NET CARBS
AVOCADO half (half of the fruit)	12g	8.5g	3.5g
BLACKBERRIES fresh (1/4 cup)	3.5g	2g	1.5g
BLACKBERRIES frozen (1/4 cup)	6g	2g	4g
BLUBERRIES frozen (1/4 cup)	5g	1g	4g
CHERRIES fresh sweet w/o pit (1/4 cup)	5g	1g	4g
CHERRIES fresh sour w/o pit (1/4 cup)	6g	1g	5g
CRANBERRIES raw and chopped (1/4 cup)	3g	1g	2g
CURRANTS fresh white and red (1/4 cup)	4g	1g	3g
GOOSEBERRIES raw (1/4 cup)	4g	1.5g	2.5g
	TOTAL	**FIBER**	**NET**

	CARB CONTENT	CONTENT	CARBS
LOGANBERRIES frozen (1/4 cup)	5g	2g	3g
MELON cantaloupe (1/4 cup)	3.5g	0.5g	3g
MELON honeydew (1/4 cup)	4g	0.5g	3.5g
RASPBERRIES fresh (1/4 cup)	4g	0.5g	3.5g
RASPBERRIES frozen (1/4 cup)	4g	2g	2g
STRAWBERRIES fresh (1/4 cup)	1.5g	0.5g	1g
STRAWBERRIES frozen (1/4 cup)	3.5g	1g	2.5g

Organ Meats

I've saved the best for last! High in fat and very nutritious, organ meats are incredible for ketosis. They are rich in vitamin A that help in reducing inflammation. They contain B-complex vitamins and protect against anemia. They also promote mitochondrial energy production and even help with fertility. Let's look at some of the most nutritious organ meats you can indulge in on a ketogenic diet.

1. Tongue

70 percent of the tongue is fatty acids. This makes it among the most tender beef cuts. In fact, there are a lot of people who enjoy its flavor more than they do steaks and ground beef. If you're a tongue beginner, it can be a little intimidating but they are actually easy to prepare and there are tons of recipes they can be used for.

2. Heart

They may not look very appetizing at first but if you the heart to give it a try, you'll be surprised to discover how tasty they are. People who've grown to like it say it's similar to the taste and texture of brisket or steak.

Hearts provide a great deal of B vitamins, zinc, iron and selenium. They are especially prized for their CoQ10 content which is very essential in promoting mitochondrial health as well as energy production. People suffering from chronic conditions can greatly benefit from this.

The most nutritious hearts are beef, venison, buffalo, and bison. Hearts are lean and muscular so they're not very high in fat. Most people like them ground. They do well when mixed with ground beef.

3. Liver

If you're looking for the most nutrient dense food on earth, this one is it! Liver is rich in retinol whether it is beef liver, chicken liver or cod liver. It also contains high amounts of bioavailable folate, B12, and choline. It's also an excellent source of zinc, iron, and selenium.

If you're a liver beginner, you may want to add it in a stew or try mixing it up with ground beef on an 80/20 ratio. This way, you barely notice it until you acquire the taste for this incredibly nutritious organ.

4. Kidney

Another nutrient-dense food, kidneys contain protein in concentrated form. You can get kidneys from lamb of beef or even chicken and turkey. Make sure you get one with its long strip fat still intact. The best ones are from grass-fed lamb or beef. They are rich in saturated fats and omega-3 fatty acids which are responsible for the organ's anti-inflammatory properties.

When it comes to flavor, the mildest ones are beef kidneys. They are most recommended for starters. For an even milder taste, you can soak them in chilled water with pink salt. Allow sitting for about two hours before you cook them. They can be boiled, braised or sautéed.

5. Spleen and SweetBreads

Also known as the pancreas and thymus, they are a delicacy. Unlike most meat that is savory, spleen and sweetbreads have a uniquely sweet flavor. They are quite high in minerals including selenium and zinc which are essential for a healthy immunity and hormonal function. They are also excellent sources of omega-3 fatty acids and protein which are anti-inflammatory.

6. Brain

Among the richest and best source of omega-3 fatty acids DHA and EPA, brain also contains neurological enhancing nutrients like phosphatidylserine and phosphatidylcholine. Brain also protects the neurological tissues against oxidative stress with its antioxidant properties.

7. Tripe and Intestines

A super source of micronutrients, tripe and intestines are an excellent way of promoting digestive health. They may be quite rubbery in texture so they have to be cooked down a while. They make a great addition to bone broth stew.

Keto-Friendly Drinks/ Beverages

During or towards ketosis, water is your best bet. But there are also quite a few more drinks you can get away with on a ketogenic diet. Although some ketogenic diet guidelines will say it's okay to drink alcohol, I strongly discourage you to. But if you can't help it, make sure you choose low to zero carbs.

	FAT CONTENT	PROTEIN CONTENT	NET CARB CONTENT
ALMOND MILK unsweetened (1 cup)	2.88g	1.55g	0g
BOUILLON/ BROTH no added sugar, not low sodium (1 cup)	0g	6.25g	0.79g
COFFEE caffeinated/ decaffeinated (1 cup)	0.05g	0.54g	0g
HEMP MILK unsweetened (1 cup)	4g	2g	1g
LEMON/ LIME JUICE (1 pc)	0.12g	0.17g	3.21g
TEA caffeinated/ decaffeinated (1 cup)	0g	0.54g	0g

Condiments and Sauces

One of the things most people hate about diet foods is the blandness of the dishes. Your keto food does not have to. However, since using a couple of condiments and sauces is out of the question, making your food tasty will require a bit of effort. The best route is to make your own but there are also a couple of keto-friendly options like the ones on this list.

CONDIMENTS/ SAUCES	FAT CONTENT	PROTEIN CONTENT	NET CARB CONTENT
ANCHO CHILI PEPPER (1 pepper)	1.4g	2g	5g
ANCHOVY PASTE (1 tbsp)	1.5g	3g	0g

CONDIMENTS/ SAUCES	FAT CONTENT	PROTEIN CONTENT	NET CARB CONTENT
CAPERS (1 tbsp)	0.07g	0.2g	0.1g
CHIPOTLE en ADOBO (2 peppers)	1g	0g	2g
CLAM JUICE (1 cup)	0g	15.8g	0g
COCONUT AMINOS (1 tsp)	0g	0g	1g
COCONUT MILK unsweetened, canned (1/2 cup)	24g	2.3g	3g
COCOA POWDER unsweetened (1 tbsp)	0.74g	1g	3g
ENCHILADA SAUCE (1/4 cup)	0g	1g	4g
FISH SAUCE (1 tsp)	0g	0.66g	0g
HORSERADISH SAUCE (1 tsp)	2.85g	0.6g	0.4g
JALAPENO CHILI PEPPER (1/2 cup)	0.33g	1.4g	5.5g
MISO PASTE (1 tbsp)	1g	2g	3g
MUSTARD DIJON (1 tsp)	0g	0g	1g
MUSTARD YELLOW (1 tsp)	0g	0g	0g
PASILLA CHILI PEPPER (1 pepper)	1.11g	0.86g	1.68g
PESTO SAUCE (1 tbsp)	5.8g	0.7g	1g
PICKAPEPPA SAUCE (1 tsp)	0g	0g	1g
PICKLE, dill or kosher (1/2 pickle)	0.07g	0.11g	0.3g
PIMENTO or ROASTED RED PEPPER (1 oz.)	0.08g	0.3g	0.9g
SALSA green, no added sugar (1 tbsp)	0g	0g	0.6g
SALSA red, no added sugar (1 tbsp)	0g	0g	1g
SERRANO CHILI PEPPER (1/2 cup)	0.23g	0.9g	1.6g
SOY SAUCE (1 tbsp)	0g	1.9g	0.9g

	FAT	PROTEIN	NET CARB
SRIRACHA (1 tsp)	0.06g	1.13g	1.15g
TABASCO or Other Hot Sauce (1 tsp)	0.04g	0.06g	0.04g
TACO SAUCE (1 tbsp)	0g	0g	2g
TAHINI sesame paste (2 tbsp)	16g	5.2g	5g
VINEGAR BALSAMIC (1 tbsp)	0g	0.8g	2.7g
VINEGAR CIDER (1 tbsp)	0g	0g	0.14g
VINEGAR RED WINE (1 tbsp)	0g	0.01g	0.04g
VINEGAR SHERRY (1 tbsp)	0g	0g	2g
VINEGAR WHITE WINE (1 tbsp)	0g	0.01g	0.12g
WASABI PASTE (1 tsp)	0g	0g	2g
WORCESTERSHIRE SAUCE (1 tbsp)	0g	0g	3.3g

Keto-Friendly Dressings

You'll probably grow some love for salads like most people on a ketogenic diet do mainly because they are the easiest to prepare. To complement your reliable green salad, consider the following dressing options. Again, be mindful of the portions. Each tablespoon can make or break your ketosis. Have a look.

DRESSINGS	FAT CONTENT	PROTEIN CONTENT	NET CARB CONTENT
BLUE CHEESE DRESSING (2 tbsp)	14g	1g	1g
CAESAR SALAD DRESSING (2 tbsp)	16g	1g	0.5g
ITALIAN DRESSING (2 tbsp)	6.2g	0.12g	3.6g
LEMON JUICE (2 tbsp)	0.07g	0.11g	2g
LIME JUICE (2 tbsp)	0.02g	0.13g	2.4g

| OIL and VINEGAR (2 tbsp) | 16g | 0g | 0.8g |
| RANCH DRESSING (2 tbsp) | 13g | 0.4g | 1.7g |

Herbs and Spices

Most traditional seasonings don't make it to the cut on a ketogenic diet. That's because most of them are made with added sugars and carbs. For flavor, you can rely on herbs and spices instead. You just have to make sure that using pure ones, not those that contain sugar. Here are a couple of herbs and spices that are keto-friendly.

BASIL	NUTMEG
CAYENNE PEPPER	OREGANO
CHILI POWDER	PARSLEY
CILANTRO	ROSEMARY
CINNAMON	SALT and PEPPER
CUMIN	THYME
LEMON/ LIME JUICE	

Sweeteners

As much as possible, you should stay away from sweeteners. They are incredibly tricky. If you must use one, you should follow these guidelines.

- Only go for sweeteners with low glycemic index. They are less likely to affect blood sugar levels. Also, they won't contribute to your daily carb consumption.
- Avoid sweeteners with sugar alcohol maltitol. They are high glycemic. It is also in your best interest to stay away from those that contain filler ingredients such as

maltodextrin and dextrose. Be careful about sweeteners that market themselves as no- or low-calorie and no- or low-sugar.

- When it comes to granulated sweeteners, every teaspoon amounts to 1g of net carbs. They more likely contain bulking agents and those can possibly incite an insulin response.

Supplements

Allow me to emphasize that supplementing is not a requirement on a ketogenic diet. They are optional. If you feel like you need the extra help, here's something to guide you and keep your keto journey going as smoothly as possible.

1. Exogenous Ketones

The main purpose of these supplements is to give your body extra ketones for energy. They may prove beneficial in the process of transitioning to ketosis. They may also help put your body back into ketosis. Exogenous ketones may be ingested in between meals or before your workout session to give you a boost of energy.

2. MCT Powders and Oils

MCT or medium chain triglyceride is a kind of fat. They are readily available fuel. That means they don't require much from your digestive system before they can be usable. MCTs can prove helpful in leading the body to start burning fat instead of carbs.

MCTs have antioxidant properties that can assist in reducing internal inflammation. They can also aid in promoting brain and heart health.

3. Collagen Protein Supplements

A type of protein, collagen is probably the most abundant in the human body. The best way to describe collagen is to compare it to a flue that holds everything in the body together.

There are other animal-based protein products but they can cause inflammation. For instance, whey and casein are allergens while egg protein can prove to be inflammatory. Collagen protein, on the other hand, is not. They are harnessed from slow and low heating in order to preserve its nutrition.

4. Micronutrient Supplements

There are a lot of vegetables and fruits that you are discouraged from eating while on a ketogenic diet. The downside is you can possibly miss out on the nutrients that can be derived from them. Micronutrient supplements offer a solution. It is packed with adequate nutrition from produce without giving you the extra carbs.

5. Keto Pre-Workout Supplements

These are made for people who like a boost of energy for their workouts while on a ketogenic diet. Energy bars and energy mixes are filled with junk. These keto-friendly pre-workout supplements, on the other hand, can provide a much-needed energy boost while keeping it clean and healthy. Aside from enhancing physical performance, they may also be beneficial in boosting cognitive performance.

In order to reach and maintain ketosis, you have to be mindful of what you put into your mouth. The source matters a lot. Keep this list in mind when it comes to planning your keto meals. They will absolutely keep you on track.

Chapter 8 - Measuring Ketosis

Let's say you put in the time and effort. How can you tell if you are indeed doing things right? How do you know you've stepped into the state of ketosis?

How to Know if You are in Ketosis?

Technically speaking, you are in the state of ketosis when your ketone levels are either at or above 0.5 mmol/L. I've mentioned different ways of measuring your ketone levels in the previous chapter. You've got the option to do a breath test, a urine test or a blood test. But are these tests necessary? The answer is a little bit more complex. Let's begin with a NO.

There are various ways to tell if you're on the right track. Your body will tell you when you are in ketosis. It will manifest as physical symptoms.

You do number 1 more often.

A natural diuretic, keto will increase your urination. Frequent visits to the bathroom can indicate you are indeed in keto.

Your mouth is dry.

Because you urinate more frequently, you lose fluids which leads to another physical symptom., increased thirst, and dry mouth. When you do feel these symptoms, you should drink plenty of water. Proper hydration will allow your body to ease in more safely to the process.

Your breath smells bad.

Unless you have bad oral hygiene, this sign is pretty huge. As the body produces and uses ketone bodies, a partial amount of these ketones are eliminated through the breath. It will be a sharp odor so there's no way you'd miss it. It may smell something like an overripe fruit. Don't worry though. This side effect is only temporary. It fades after a while. Give it a week or so.

You feel less hungry and more energized!

Let me make this one thing clear. Ketosis won't magically energize you. As with anything else in this life, you got to pay your dues first. You will likely feel worse before you feel better. After the phase we refer to as "keto flu," you will begin to feel much better, way better than you have before.

You will get past the hunger pains. And you will eventually have a clearer state of mind. You will feel more energized and ready to take over the world or something like that.

Other Side Effects of Ketosis and How to Prevent Them

While we are on the topic of signs, let's look at the other common side effects of ketosis you should watch out for.

1. Dizziness and Drowsiness

This occurs as a result of the loss of minerals. As your body eliminates water, some minerals are flushed out too. As a result, you may feel fatigued, lightheaded and dizzy.

To avoid this or at least reduce the severity, you can consume more foods that are high in potassium like leafy green vegetables, broccoli, meat, poultry and fish, dairy and avocados. You can also try a salty broth or simply add salt in your drinking water.

2. Low Blood Sugar

This happens a lot to those who are used to having a higher carb intake. It's a withdrawal symptom from all the sugar. It happens temporarily but you probably should prepare yourself for some shaky and hungry moments, at least until your body has fully adapted to the change in your diet.

3. Sugar Cravings

This is probably among the most challenging side effects. And it can be worse during the transition period. But when you're craving for chocolate, it's just your body telling you it needs magnesium which can be fixed by eating nuts and seeds instead. Here are other ideas on how to combat those nasty cravings.

4. Diarrhea or Constipation

While the digestive system tries to adapt, a case of either diarrhea or constipation may occur. To combat these side effects, drink plenty of water. You may want to take it easy on nuts and dairy in the meantime too.

5. Muscle Cramps

With the loss of minerals, muscle cramps occur. Proper hydration is the key to relief and prevention.

6. Sleep Issues

This may occur as a result of low insulin and serotonin levels or you're consuming foods that are high in histamines. To help relieve the issue, cut back on your consumption of eggs, bacon, avocado, and cheese. They contain histamines which can possibly cause sleep problems. Also, up your dosage of low carb vegetables for relief.

7. Heart Palpitations

This is a common side effect experienced by people with a normally low blood pressure. I cannot emphasize the importance of salt and water further. Drink up!

8. Flu-Like Symptoms

This is what they refer to as keto flu. It usually occurs in the first 2-4 days of getting into the diet. Symptoms may include headaches, tiredness, lethargy, brain fog, and irritability.

Can You Possibly Avoid These Side Effects?

You may not completely avoid them but you can absolutely reduce the symptoms and find relief. There are three major things to do. Learn it by heart and make it your motto especially during the transition period.

- Drink plenty of water!
- Put salt in your food or in your water!
- Eat enough fat!

What is ketoacidosis?

Ketoacidosis is as bad as it sounds. In this condition, the ketone levels reach abnormally high rates which lead to poisoning. It quickly develops and is likely to occur within 24 hours. Among the early symptoms include:

-rapid breathing or shortness of breath

-nausea and vomiting

-more frequent urination

-smelly breath

-dry mouth and excessive thirst

-dry skin

-difficulty concentrating

-abdominal pain

Should you worry about ketoacidosis as you get into the keto diet? This condition is most common among type 1 diabetes patients who are unable to produce insulin. It may sometimes occur in type 2 diabetes but it rarely does. Unless you suffer from these conditions, there's no reason for you to panic. In any case, there are home kits available to help you monitor your ketone levels.

Testing Blood Ketones

These physical side effects will let you know you are doing things right. But to find out exactly what level you're at, you will probably need to get one of those tests.

If you happen to get a blood ketone test, it can accurately tell you whether or not you're in ketosis yet and which level you're at exactly.

Light Ketosis: 0.5 mmol/L – 0.8 mmol/L

Medium Ketosis: 0.9 mmol/L – 1.4 mmol/L

Deep Ketosis: 1.5 mmol/L – 3.0 mmol/L

Most people step into light ketosis in 2 to 3 days from the diet alone. It will take much longer to reach a deep ketosis. It usually occurs after 2 to 3 weeks of following the diet.

Ketosis Best for...

- People with neurological conditions like Parkinson's and Alzheimer's or behavioral disorders such as Autism
- Individuals suffering from any of these conditions: obesity, diabetes, and non-alcoholic fatty liver disease.
- Children with epilepsy

Or if you are a healthy individual who wants to enhance your cognitive function, boost your energy level and improve your overall health, you can obviously benefit from ketosis too.

Ketosis is NOT Recommended for...

Ketosis is not a magical panacea and it should not be treated as such. With this said, there are some who may not benefit as much from ketosis.

- Athletes in general, who rely on high bursts of performance
- People with genetic mutations that will prevent them from efficiently burning ketones and possibly, impair their body's ability to buffer ketone acidity

Fortunately, such genetic mutations are rare. To be on the safe side, if you're suffering from a health condition, it is best to seek supervision from a medical professional before getting into the diet.

Chapter 9 - Shopping List and Guidelines

We've talked about the many wonderful benefits of ketosis in full detail. It sounds challenging and exciting and you can hardly wait to get started. Wait. How do you begin exactly? Don't worry, I got you.

To help make the process suited to you, I suggest you follow these steps.

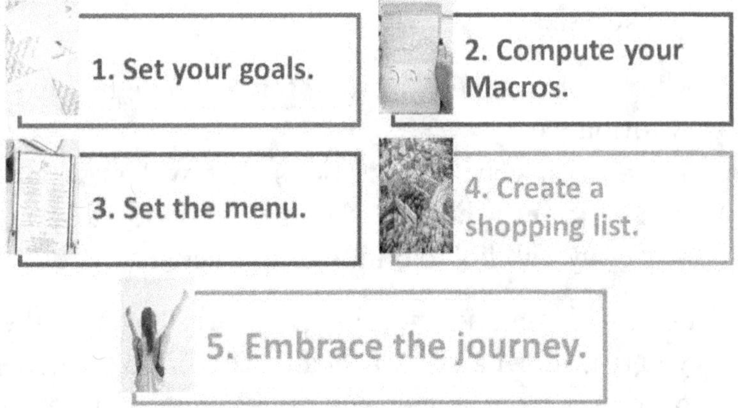

Set your goals.

You want this for a reason so what is that reason? Do you want to save yourself from disease? Do you want your overall health improved? Do you want to be in a much better shape and feel amazing about your body? Whatever your goals are, state it clearly. Do you want to maintain your current weight or shed some?

Compute your Macros.

Whether your goal is disease prevention or mainly weight loss, your weight will be affected. Set your daily target for the following: calories, fat, protein, and carbs.

You see this ketogenic pie all the time but how do you arrive at those percentages?

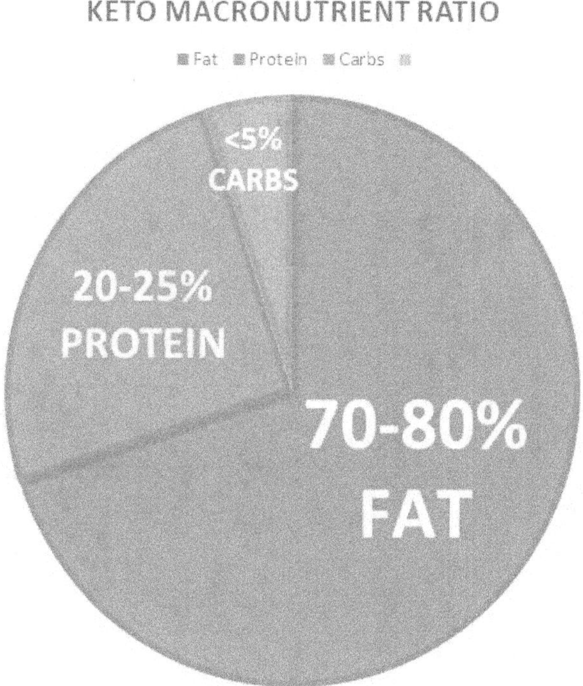

Let's start with calories. Although calorie counting is not the main focus here, you should at least be mindful of your calorie digits. Remember this computation from the earlier chapters.

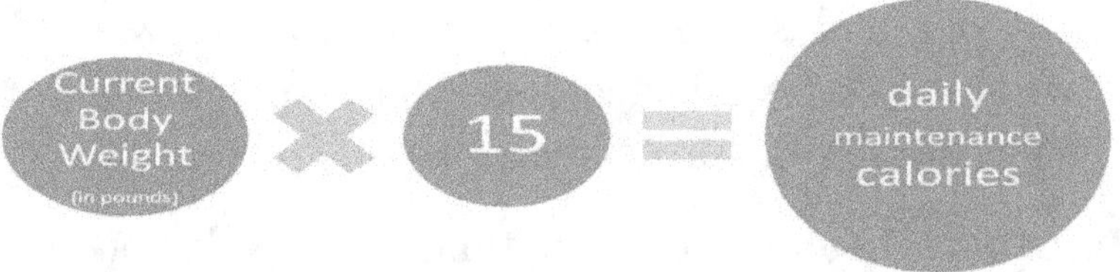

If you want to lose weight, you will have to go below the daily maintenance caloric requirement. Now that we have the calorie portion cleared up, let's think about carbs. Limit your carb intake to 20-50g of daily net carbs or make sure you are within 5% of your daily calorie intake.

As for protein, you can use this equation to determine your ideal range.

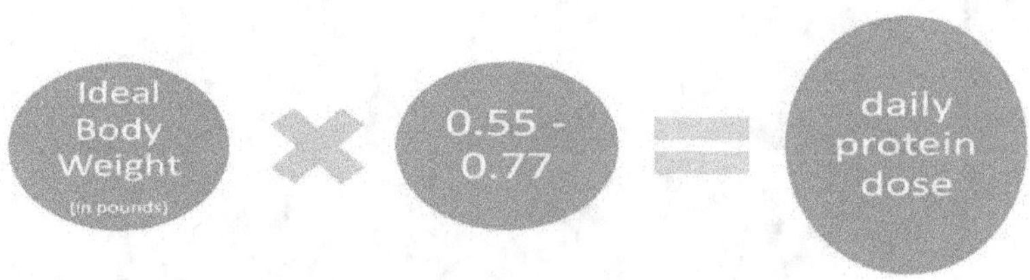

And the rest should consist of fat. The ketogenic diet sets a range for fat consumption at 70-80% of your daily calorie allowance. Make sure you're hitting the mark.

Set the menu.

Based on your calculated daily macros, you are now ready to plan your meals. I've prepared for you a sample meal plan for 21 days. If they aren't within your target daily macros, feel free to make changes. The recipes are flexible enough to make room for adjustments.

As you get into the process, I'm sure you will become more adventurous in your meal choices. It's an opportunity for you to explore so go for it.

When creating your menu, I suggest that you do it on a weekly basis. Not everyone has the time to make the effort in the kitchen on a daily basis. Consider recipes that you can make a big batch of so you have enough stash on days you can't wear the apron.

Create a shopping list.

Remember there are rules to live by on a ketogenic diet. Making a list of your ingredients based on the meal plan you've created will help you further assess whether or not you're keeping within your limits. I'm including here a sample shopping list with all the keto-friendly food items.

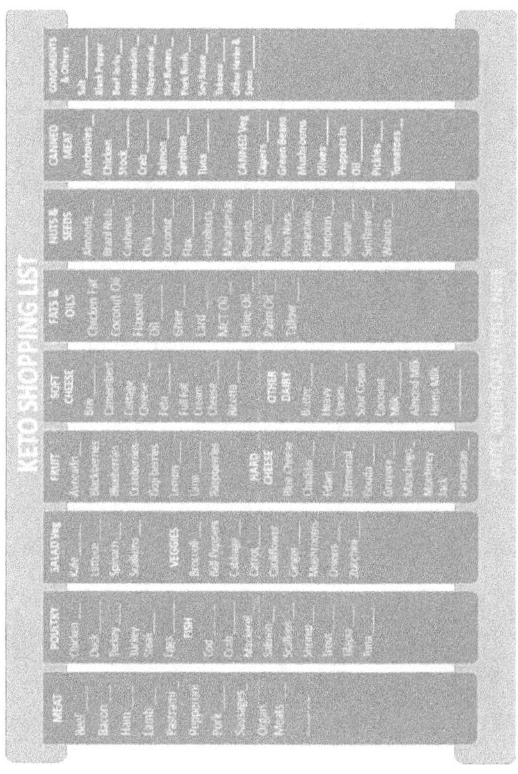

Embrace the journey!

Finally, you should go ahead and embrace the journey. There will be ups and downs so brace yourself. In the end, you will find what you're looking for. Just go for it!

Chapter 10 – 21-Day Meal Plan

To make your keto journey a little easier, I've prepared a sample meal plan here. You will find the shopping list in the previous chapter.

Like I mentioned, it is important to set your daily calorie goal beforehand. It will guide you through the entire process of choosing and planning your meals.

WEEK 1 MEAL PLAN

To make things as simple as possible for you, I've prepared only 9 recipes for you to learn in the first week. You can cook them in a big batch before the week starts to save time. Since your body will still be adjusting, I've set daily calorie allowance to a range of 1500-1850 calories. You can adjust the meal plan according to your goal but I suggest that you take it easy on your first week.

You will notice that the net carbs on some days are below 20g. If you feel like you need to keep at a 20-50g allowance, feel free to get some snacks in order to fill the gaps.

Day One

BREAKFAST	MACROS
1 cup of tea or coffee mixed with MCT oil powder 4 slices of fried bacon in 1 tablespoon of butter Turkey sausage frittata, 1 serving	Calories: 572 FAT: 49.7g PROTEIN: 24.7g CARBS: 5.5g
LUNCH	
Bone broth, 1 serving Half head of romaine lettuce leaves Quarter pound ground beef	Calories: 500.5 FAT: 38g PROTEIN: 26.25g CARBS: 1.5g
DINNER	
Keto Mayo, 1 serving Celeriac Oven Fries, 1 serving Portobello Cheeseburger, 1 serving	Calories: 539 FAT: 40.2g PROTEIN: 31.1g CARBS: 13.1g
DESSERT/ SNACK	
Fat Bombs with Macadamia Nuts	Calories: 198 FAT: 33.8g PROTEIN: 1.6g CARBS: 1.8g

Total Macros for the Day

FAT	PROTEIN	CARBS	Calories
161.7g	83.65	22g	1,809.5

Day Two

BREAKFAST	MACROS
1 cup of tea or coffee mixed with MCT oil powder Choco Pancakes served with Blueberry Butter, 1 serving	Calories: 611 FAT: 57g PROTEIN: 26.6g CARBS: 11.5g

LUNCH	
Crispy "Fried" Chicken with Salad, 1 serving	Calories: 575 FAT: 36.4g PROTEIN: 55g CARBS: 8.1g

DINNER	
4 ounces of grilled ribeye steak in 2 tablespoons of butter 2 cups of mixed leafy greens served with 1 tablespoon of avocado oil plus salt as dressing	Calories: 636 FAT: 62g PROTEIN: 20g CARBS: 1g

Total Macros for the Day

FAT	PROTEIN	CARBS	Calories
155.4g	101.6	20.6g	1,822

Day Three

BREAKFAST	MACROS
1 cup of tea or coffee mixed with MCT oil powder 4 slices of fried bacon in 1 tablespoon of butter Fat Bombs with Macadamia Nuts	Calories: 530 FAT: 66.8g PROTEIN: 9.6g CARBS: 1.8g
LUNCH	
Keto Mayo, 1 serving Celeriac Oven Fries, 1 serving Portobello Cheeseburger, 1 serving	Calories: 539 FAT: 40.2g PROTEIN: 31.1g CARBS: 13.1g
DINNER	
Bone Broth, 1 serving Turkey Sausage Frittata 1 serving Keto Mayo Dip, 1 serving	Calories: 434 FAT: 35g PROTEIN: 23.1g CARBS: 6.5g

Total Macros for the Day

FAT	PROTEIN	CARBS	Calories
142g	63.8g	21.4g	1,503

Day Four

BREAKFAST	MACROS
1 cup of tea or coffee mixed with MCT oil powder Choco Pancakes served with Blueberry Butter, 1 serving	Calories: 611 FAT: 57g PROTEIN: 26.6g CARBS: 11.5g
LUNCH	
Bone broth, 1 serving Half head of romaine lettuce leaves Quarter pound ground beef	Calories: 500.5 FAT: 38g PROTEIN: 26.25g CARBS: 1.5g
DINNER	
4 ounces of grilled ribeye steak in 2 tablespoons of butter 2 cups of mixed leafy greens served with 1 tablespoon of avocado oil plus salt as dressing	Calories: 636 FAT: 62g PROTEIN: 20g CARBS: 1g

Total Macros for the Day

FAT	PROTEIN	CARBS	Calories
157g	72.85	13.5g	1,747.5

Day Five

BREAKFAST	MACROS
1 cup of tea or coffee mixed with MCT oil powder 4 slices of fried bacon in 1 tablespoon of butter Turkey sausage frittata, 1 serving	Calories: 572 FAT: 49.7g PROTEIN: 24.7g CARBS: 5.5g
LUNCH	
White Turkey Chili, 1 serving 2 cups of mixed leafy greens 1 tablespoon of olive oil as dressing	Calories: 568 FAT: 44.5g PROTEIN: 28.8g CARBS: 5.5g
DINNER	
Keto Mayo, 1 serving Celeriac Oven Fries, 1 serving Portobello Cheeseburger, 1 serving	Calories: 539 FAT: 40.2g PROTEIN: 31.1g CARBS: 13.1g
DESSERT/ SNACK	
Fat Bombs with Macadamia Nuts	Calories: 198 FAT: 33.8g PROTEIN: 1.6g CARBS: 1.8g

Total Macros for the Day

FAT	PROTEIN	CARBS	Calories
168.2g	86.2	25.9g	1,877

Day Six

BREAKFAST	MACROS
1 cup of tea or coffee mixed with MCT oil powder Choco Pancakes served with Blueberry Butter, 1 serving	Calories: 611 FAT: 57g PROTEIN: 26.6g CARBS: 11.5g
LUNCH	
4 ounces of grilled ribeye steak in 2 tablespoons of butter 2 cups of mixed leafy greens served with 1 tablespoon of avocado oil plus salt as dressing	Calories: 636 FAT: 62g PROTEIN: 20g CARBS: 1g
DINNER	
Crispy "Fried" Chicken, 1 serving 2 cups of mixed leafy greens served with 1 tablespoon of avocado oil plus salt as dressing	Calories: 575 FAT: 36.4g PROTEIN: 55g CARBS: 8.1g

Total Macros for the Day

FAT	PROTEIN	CARBS	Calories
155.4g	101.6	20.6g	1,822

Day Seven

BREAKFAST	MACROS
1 cup of tea or coffee mixed with MCT oil powder 4 slices of fried bacon in 1 tablespoon of butter Fat Bombs with Macadamia Nuts	Calories: 530 FAT: 66.8g PROTEIN: 9.6g CARBS: 1.8g

LUNCH	MACROS
White Turkey Chili, 1 serving 2 cups of mixed leafy greens 1 tablespoon of olive oil as dressing	Calories: 568 FAT: 44.5g PROTEIN: 28.8g CARBS: 5.5g

DINNER	MACROS
Bone Broth, 1 serving Turkey Sausage Frittata 1 serving Keto Mayo Dip, 1 serving	Calories: 434 FAT: 35g PROTEIN: 23.1g CARBS: 6.5g

Total Macros for the Day

FAT	PROTEIN	CARBS	Calories
146.3g	61.5g	13.8g	1,532

WEEK 2 MEAL PLAN

At this point, your body is still adjusting but you may begin to get used to the new diet. I've added a couple more recipes for you to learn and switch around throughout the week. For the purpose of dieting for weight loss, the daily calorie allowance for the second week is set to a range of 1300 to 1550 calories.

Day Eight

BREAKFAST	MACROS
1 cup of tea or coffee mixed with MCT oil powder 4 slices of fried bacon in 1 tablespoon of butter Fat Bombs with Macadamia Nuts	Calories: 530 FAT: 66.8g PROTEIN: 9.6g CARBS: 1.8g
LUNCH	
Keto Mayo, 1 serving Celeriac Oven Fries, 1 serving Portobello Cheeseburger, 1 serving	Calories: 539 FAT: 40.2g PROTEIN: 31.1g CARBS: 13.1g
DINNER	
Bone Broth, 1 serving Turkey Sausage Frittata 1 serving	Calories: 310 FAT: 20.7g PROTEIN: 22.7g CARBS: 6.5g

Total Macros for the Day

FAT	PROTEIN	CARBS	Calories
127.7g	63.4g	21.4g	1,379

Day Nine

BREAKFAST	MACROS
1 cup of tea or coffee mixed with MCT oil powder Keto Brunch Spread, 1 serving	Calories: 528 FAT: 57g PROTEIN: 17g CARBS: 3g
LUNCH White Turkey Chili, 1 serving 2 cups of mixed leafy greens 1 tablespoon of olive oil as dressing	Calories: 568 FAT: 44.5g PROTEIN: 28.8g CARBS: 5.5g
DINNER Bone Broth, 1 serving Portobello Cheeseburger, 1 serving	Calories: 406 FAT: 26.8g PROTEIN: 33.1g CARBS: 10g

Total Macros for the Day

FAT	PROTEIN	CARBS	Calories
128.3g	78.9	18.5g	1,502

Day Ten

BREAKFAST	MACROS
1 cup of tea or coffee mixed with MCT oil powder Choco Pancakes served with Blueberry Butter, 1 serving	Calories: 611 FAT: 57g PROTEIN: 26.6g CARBS: 11.5g

LUNCH	MACROS
Zesty Chicken Taco, 1 serving Blue Cheese Dressing, 1 tbsp	Calories: 360 FAT: 36g PROTEIN: 31g, CARBS: 6g

DINNER	MACROS
Crispy "Fried" Chicken, 1 serving 2 cups of mixed leafy greens served with 1 tablespoon of avocado oil plus salt as dressing	Calories: 575 FAT: 36.4g PROTEIN: 55g CARBS: 8.1g

Total Macros for the Day

FAT	PROTEIN	CARBS	Calories
129.4g	112.6	25.6g	1,546

Day Eleven

BREAKFAST	MACROS
1 cup of tea or coffee mixed with MCT oil powder Keto Brunch Spread, 1 serving	Calories: 528 FAT: 57g PROTEIN: 17g CARBS: 3g
LUNCH	
4 ounces of grilled ribeye steak in 2 tablespoons of butter 2 cups of mixed leafy greens served with 1 tablespoon of avocado oil plus salt as dressing	Calories: 636 FAT: 62g PROTEIN: 20g CARBS: 1g
DINNER	
Shrimp Stacks, 1 serving	Calories: 289 FAT: 21.8g PROTEIN: 12.3g CARBS: 14.2g

Total Macros for the Day

FAT	PROTEIN	CARBS	Calories
140.8g	49.3	18.2g	1,453

Day Twelve

BREAKFAST

1 cup of tea or coffee mixed with MCT oil powder
4 slices of fried bacon in 1 tablespoon of butter
Turkey sausage frittata, 1 serving

MACROS

Calories: 572
FAT: 49.7g
PROTEIN: 24.7g
CARBS: 5.5g

LUNCH

Keto Mayo, 1 serving
Celeriac Oven Fries, 1 serving
Portobello Cheeseburger, 1 serving

Calories: 539
FAT: 40.2g
PROTEIN: 31.1g
CARBS: 13.1g

DINNER

Zesty Chicken Taco, 1 serving
Blue Cheese Dressing, 1 tbsp

Calories: 360
FAT: 36g
PROTEIN: 31g
CARBS: 6g

Total Macros for the Day

FAT	PROTEIN	CARBS	Calories
125.9g	86.8g	24.6g	1,471

Day Thirteen

BREAKFAST   MACROS

1 cup of tea or coffee mixed with MCT oil powder Keto Brunch Spread, 1 serving	Calories: 528 FAT: 57g PROTEIN: 17g CARBS: 3g

LUNCH

White Turkey Chili, 1 serving 2 cups of mixed leafy greens 1 tablespoon of olive oil as dressing	Calories: 568 FAT: 44.5g PROTEIN: 28.8g CARBS: 5.5g

DINNER

Bone Broth, 1 serving Portobello Cheeseburger, 1 serving	Calories: 406 FAT: 26.8g PROTEIN: 33.1g CARBS: 10g

Total Macros for the Day

FAT	PROTEIN	CARBS	Calories
128.3g	78.9	18.5g	1,502

Day Fourteen

BREAKFAST	MACROS
1 cup of tea or coffee mixed with MCT oil powder 4 slices of fried bacon in 1 tablespoon of butter Fat Bombs with Macadamia Nuts	Calories: 530 FAT: 66.8g PROTEIN: 9.6g CARBS: 1.8g

LUNCH	MACROS
White Turkey Chili, 1 serving 2 cups of mixed leafy greens 1 tablespoon of olive oil as dressing	Calories: 568 FAT: 44.5g PROTEIN: 28.8g CARBS: 5.5g

DINNER	MACROS
Bone Broth, 1 serving Turkey Sausage Frittata 1 serving Keto Mayo Dip, 1 serving	Calories: 434 FAT: 35g PROTEIN: 23.1g CARBS: 6.5g

Total Macros for the Day

FAT	PROTEIN	CARBS	Calories
146.3g	61.5g	13.8g	1,532

WEEK 3 MEAL PLAN

Kudos for holding on. By now, you should be familiar with the recipes. In the third week, we're maintaining the daily calorie allowance to 1300- 1550 calories.

Day Fifteen

BREAKFAST	MACROS
1 cup of tea or coffee mixed with MCT oil powder Keto Brunch Spread, 1 serving	Calories: 528 FAT: 57g PROTEIN: 17g CARBS: 3g
LUNCH Shrimp Stacks, 1 serving	Calories: 289 FAT: 21.8g PROTEIN: 12.3g CARBS: 14.2g
DINNER 4 ounces of grilled ribeye steak in 2 tablespoons of butter 2 cups of mixed leafy greens served with 1 tablespoon of avocado oil plus salt as dressing	Calories: 636 FAT: 62g PROTEIN: 20g CARBS: 1g

Total Macros for the Day

FAT	PROTEIN	CARBS	Calories
140.8g	49.3	18.2g	1,453

Day Sixteen

BREAKFAST	MACROS
1 cup of tea or coffee mixed with MCT oil powder 4 slices of fried bacon in 1 tablespoon of butter Fat Bombs with Macadamia Nuts	Calories: 530 FAT: 66.8g PROTEIN: 9.6g CARBS: 1.8g

LUNCH	
Keto Mayo, 1 serving Celeriac Oven Fries, 1 serving Portobello Cheeseburger, 1 serving	Calories: 539 FAT: 40.2g PROTEIN: 31.1g CARBS: 13.1g

DINNER	
Bone Broth, 1 serving Turkey Sausage Frittata 1 serving	Calories: 310 FAT: 20.7g PROTEIN: 22.7g CARBS: 6.5g

Total Macros for the Day

FAT	PROTEIN	CARBS	Calories
127.7g	63.4g	21.4g	1,379

Day Seventeen

BREAKFAST	MACROS
1 cup of tea or coffee mixed with MCT oil powder Crispy Bacon wrapped in Asparagus, 5 bundles Keto Mayo Dipping	Calories: 354 FAT: 34.3g PROTEIN: 15.4g CARBS: 0g
LUNCH	
Bone broth, 1 serving Half head of romaine lettuce leaves Quarter pound ground beef	Calories: 500.5 FAT: 38g PROTEIN: 26.25g CARBS: 1.5g
DINNER	
Shrimp Stacks, 1 serving	Calories: 289 FAT: 21.8g PROTEIN: 12.3g CARBS: 14.2g
DESSERT/ SNACK	
Fat Bombs with Macadamia Nuts	Calories: 198 FAT: 33.8g PROTEIN: 1.6g CARBS: 1.8g

Total Macros for the Day

FAT	PROTEIN	CARBS	Calories
127.9g	43.25g	17.5g	1,341.5

Day Eighteen

BREAKFAST	MACROS
1 cup of tea or coffee mixed with MCT oil powder 4 slices of fried bacon in 1 tablespoon of butter Turkey sausage frittata, 1 serving	Calories: 572 FAT: 49.7g PROTEIN: 24.7g CARBS: 5.5g

LUNCH	
Crispy "Fried" Chicken with Salad, 1 serving Blue Cheese Dressing, 1 tbsp	Calories: 595 FAT: 50.4g PROTEIN: 56g CARBS: 9.1g

DINNER	
Zesty Chicken Taco, 1 serving Blue Cheese Dressing, 1 tbsp	Calories: 360 FAT: 36g PROTEIN: 31g CARBS: 6g

Total Macros for the Day

FAT	PROTEIN	CARBS	Calories
136.1g	111.7g	20.6g	1,527

Day Nineteen

BREAKFAST

MACROS

1 cup of tea or coffee mixed with MCT oil powder
4 slices of fried bacon in 1 tablespoon of butter
Fat Bombs with Macadamia Nuts

Calories: 530
FAT: 66.8g
PROTEIN: 9.6g
CARBS: 1.8g

LUNCH

White Turkey Chili, 1 serving
2 cups of mixed leafy greens
1 tablespoon of olive oil as dressing

Calories: 568
FAT: 44.5g
PROTEIN: 28.8g
CARBS: 5.5g

DINNER

Bone Broth, 1 serving
Turkey Sausage Frittata 1 serving
Keto Mayo Dip, 1 serving

Calories: 434
FAT: 35g
PROTEIN: 23.1g
CARBS: 6.5g

Total Macros for the Day

FAT	PROTEIN	CARBS	Calories
146.3g	61.5g	13.8g	1,532

Day Twenty

BREAKFAST	MACROS
1 cup of tea or coffee mixed with MCT oil powder Keto Brunch Spread, 1 serving	Calories: 528 FAT: 57g PROTEIN: 17g CARBS: 3g
LUNCH	
4 ounces of grilled ribeye steak in 2 tablespoons of butter 2 cups of mixed leafy greens served with 1 tablespoon of avocado oil plus salt as dressing	Calories: 636 FAT: 62g PROTEIN: 20g CARBS: 1g
DINNER	
Shrimp Stacks, 1 serving	Calories: 289 FAT: 21.8g PROTEIN: 12.3g CARBS: 14.2g

Total Macros for the Day

FAT	PROTEIN	CARBS	Calories
140.8g	49.3	18.2g	1,453

Day Twenty One

BREAKFAST	MACROS
1 cup of tea or coffee mixed with MCT oil powder 4 slices of fried bacon in 1 tablespoon of butter Fat Bombs with Macadamia Nuts	Calories: 530 FAT: 66.8g PROTEIN: 9.6g CARBS: 1.8g
LUNCH Keto Mayo, 1 serving Celeriac Oven Fries, 1 serving Portobello Cheeseburger, 1 serving	Calories: 539 FAT: 40.2g PROTEIN: 31.1g CARBS: 13.1g
DINNER Bone Broth, 1 serving Turkey Sausage Frittata 1 serving	Calories: 310 FAT: 20.7g PROTEIN: 22.7g CARBS: 6.5g

Total Macros for the Day

FAT	PROTEIN	CARBS	Calories
127.7g	63.4g	21.4g	1,379

Chapter 11 - Easy KETO Recipes for Beginners

Turkey Sausage Frittata

Total Time	40 minutes	Fat	16.7g
Servings	4	Protein	16.7g
Calories per Serving	240	Carbs	5.5g

Ingredients:

1 teaspoon of butter

1/2 teaspoon of black pepper

1/2 teaspoon of pink Himalayan salt

1/2 cup of sour cream

6 whole eggs

1 bell pepper (green or red)

6 ounces of ground turkey breakfast sausage

Directions:

1. Preheat the oven to 350 degrees Fahrenheit.

2. Crack the eggs into the blender. Season with salt and pepper. Add sour cream. Blend for 30 seconds and set it aside.

3. Place a skillet under medium heat and add butter.

4. Cut bell pepper into strips and toss into the skillet. Sauté the bell pepper strips for 6 minutes or until brown and tender. Take them out of the skillet and set aside.

5. Toss the turkey sausage into the skillet and stir. Cook for 8 minutes or until brown. Flatten the meat and add the bell pepper strips back in on top of the meat. Make sure the strips are evenly distributed before adding the egg mixture over it.

6. Turn off the heat and put the skillet into the oven. Bake it for half an hour.

Optional: Add a sprinkle of shredded cheddar (2 ounces) over the frittata before removing it from the oven.

Bone Broth

Total Time	24-48 hours	Fat	4g
Servings	6 cups	Protein	6g
Calories per Serving	70 per cup	Carbs	1g

Ingredients:

3 pieces of bay leaves

2 tablespoons of apple cider vinegar

1 teaspoon of salt

2 teaspoons of turmeric

1 whole lemon

2 tablespoons of peppercorns

10 cups filtered water

4 pounds of pastured animal bones

Directions:

1. Preheat the oven to 400 degrees Fahrenheit.

2. Arrange the bones on a sheet pan. Season with salt and roast seasoned bones for about 45 minutes.

3. Put the roasted bones in a slow cooker or electric pressure cooker.

4. Add bay leaves, water, apple cider vinegar, and peppercorns. Cook the broth on low for about 24 or up to 48 hours. If you're using a pressure cooker, cook it on high for about 2 hours and slow cook on low for about 12 hours.

5. After the cooking time, strain the broth and discard the bones, peppercorns and bay leaves.

6. Store the bone broth in mason jars. 1 mason jar can accommodate 2 cups of broth. This makes around 6 cups.

7. Add 1 teaspoon of turmeric to each jar with 1 or 2 lemon slices.

8. Store the jar in the fridge. Consume within 5 days. Simmer to heat the broth.

Keto Mayo

Total Time	10 minutes	Fat	14.3g
Servings	1 cup	Protein	0.4g
Serving Size	1 tbsp per serving	Carbs	0g
Calories per Serving	124		

Ingredients:

1/4 teaspoon of pink Himalayan salt

2 teaspoons of apple cider vinegar

1 cup of olive oil

1 whole egg

Directions:

1. Let the egg reach room temperature. If you're taking it out of the fridge, wait for 2 hours before starting. Separate the yolk from the egg white. Discard the egg white.

2. Put the egg yolk in a small container where an immersion blender can fit in. Add salt, apple cider vinegar and olive oil in the container.

3. Use the immersion blender to blend the ingredients. Put the immersion blender at the bottom while off. Hold it down and turn on. Blend for about 30 seconds or until you get a perfect mayonnaise consistency.

4. Turn off the immersion blender. To emulsify the mayonnaise, pull the immersion blender at the top of the mixture, turn it on and move it down towards the bottom of the container. Continue to do this for about 3 or 4 times and turn the blender off.

Celeriac Oven Fries

Total Time	70 minutes	Fat	9.8g
Servings	2	Protein	1.5g
Calories per Serving	124	Carbs	9g

Ingredients:

1 small celeriac root

1 1/2 tablespoons of coconut oil

1 teaspoon of bagel seasoning

Directions:

1. Preheat the oven to 400 degrees Fahrenheit.

2. Remove the bottom of the celeriac along with its roots. Peel the round portion. Slice and cut into strips.

3. Add a little lemon to water. Soak the fries.

4. Drain the fries and dry. Season the fries and add coconut oil. Toss.

5. Spread the fries on a sheet pan. Place in the oven to bake for about 30 minutes. Turn it off. Allow sitting for 10 minutes.

6. Remove sheet pan from the oven and shake the fries. Serve with mayo dipping.

Portobello Cheeseburger

Total Time	20 minutes	Fat	22.8g
Servings	6	Protein	29.1g
Calories per Serving	336	Net Carbs	4g

Ingredients:

6 slices of cheddar cheese

6 caps of Portobello mushroom, stems removed, rinsed and dabbed dried

1 tablespoon of avocado oil

1 teaspoon of black pepper

1 teaspoon of pink Himalayan salt

1 tablespoon of Worcestershire sauce

1 pound of ground beef

Directions:

1. Mix the beef with Worcestershire sauce and seasonings in a bowl.

2. Make burger patties from the mixture.

3. Heat avocado oil in a pan over medium heat. Cook each side of the mushroom caps for 3 to 4 minutes. Remove from pan.

4. Cook each side of the burger patties in the pan for 4 to 5 minutes or until done.

5. Put cheese on top of burger patties. Cover the pan to melt the cheese.

6. Lay the cheeseburger on top of one cap. Garnish and top it off with another mushroom cap.

Fat Bomb with Macadamia Nuts

Total Time	40 minutes	Fat	16.9g
Servings	6 cup	Protein	0.8g
Calories per Serving	99	Carbs	1.9g

Ingredients:

A pinch of salt

12 pieces of macadamia nuts

1 teaspoon of vanilla extract

2 tablespoons of sweetener

2 tablespoons of unsweetened cocoa powder

1/3 cup of refined coconut oil at room temperature

Directions:

1. Mix the vanilla extract, sweetener, cocoa powder and coconut oil in a bowl. Whisk them together until smooth.

2. Place a parchment paper on a small container, not bigger than 4x6. Pour the mixture into the container. Using a spatula, spread it thinly and evenly.

3. Pour the macadamia nuts over the mixture. Sprinkle with some salt.

4. Freeze the mixture for 20 minutes. When ready, cut them into 6 squares.

Choco Pancakes served with Blueberry Butter

Total Time	23 minutes	Fat	50g
Servings	2	Protein	26.6g
Calories per Serving	611	Carbs	11.5g

Ingredients:

A pinch of salt

3 tablespoons of wild blueberries, frozen

2 tablespoons of gold butter for the batter

1 tablespoon of gold butter for cooking

1/2 teaspoon of baking soda

1/4 scant cup of coconut flour

2 tablespoons of MCT oil or plain coconut oil

4 large whole eggs

Directions:

1. Place a large skillet over medium heat.

2. Mix the oil, eggs, flour, baking soda and salt in a bowl. Whisk until batter is thick.

3. Add butter into skillet. When butter melts, pour batter into the skillet. Cook each side for 4 to 5 minutes. Remove from heat

4. Pour the blueberries in a sauce pot. Cook them until thawed. Wait until the fluid simmers then add butter. Mix and mash the mixture until blueberries are softened. Pour the syrup over the pancake.

Crispy "Fried" Chicken

Total Time	40 minutes	Fat	27g
Servings	4	Protein	33g
Calories per Serving	463	Carbs	7g

Ingredients:

1 pound or 8 pieces of chicken thighs, boneless and skinless

1 teaspoon of dried Italian herbs

1 teaspoon of black pepper

1 teaspoon of Himalayan salt

1/2 cup of sesame seeds

1 cup of sunflower seeds

2 tablespoons of avocado oil

Directions:

1. Preheat your oven to 425 degrees Fahrenheit.

2. Use avocado oil to grease sheet pan.

3. Grind the seeds and mix with the seasonings.

4. Pour the seasoning mix into a big container with a lid or a freezer bag. Add the chicken one at a time. Shake until chicken thigh is well coated. Place it on the greased sheet pan. Do the same for the rest of the chicken.

5. Roast the chicken for 30 minutes, each side for 15 minutes.

White Turkey Chili

Total Time	20 minutes	Fat	30.5g
Servings	5	Protein	28.8g
Calories per Serving	388	Carbs	5.5g

Ingredients:

1 teaspoon each of the following seasonings: ground black pepper, salt, garlic powder, celery, and thyme

1 tablespoon of mustard

2 cups of heavy cream or coconut milk, full fat

2 garlic cloves

1/2 onion

2 tablespoons of coconut oil

2 cups of cauliflower rice

1 pound of ground turkey (pork, lamb or beef)

Directions:

1. Heat coconut oil in a pot.

2. Mince garlic and onion and add to the pot. Stir and cook for 2-3 minutes.

3. Add ground meat, break up using a spatula. Continue to stir until the meat is crumbled.

4. Add seasoning mix and cauliflower rice. Stir them well.

5. When the meat turns brown, pour the coconut milk into the pot. Reduce the heat and simmer for 5-8 minutes. Stir constantly until desired thickness is achieved.

Optional: You may also add shredded cheese if you want the sauce to be extra thick. Then, add any of the following as toppings: hot sauce, cherry tomatoes, bacon, jalapenos or avocados.

Keto Brunch Spread

Total Time	30 minutes	Fat	38g
Servings	4	Protein	17g
Calories per Serving	426	Carbs	3g

Ingredients:

12 slices of bacon, pastured and sugar-free

24 asparagus spears, trimmed an inch from the bottom

4 whole eggs

Directions:

1. Preheat oven to 400 degrees Fahrenheit.

2. Take two spears of asparagus and wrap a slice of bacon around them. Pull the bacon gently as you wrap the asparagus from bottom up. Place the wrapped asparagus on a sheet pan. Do the same for the rest of the asparagus.

3. Put the sheet pan into the oven. The timer should be set at 20 minutes.

4. In the meantime, bring a pot of water to boil. When boiling, put the eggs in. Set a timer for 6 minutes.

5. Have a bowl filled with ice water ready. After 6 minutes, take the eggs out of the boiling water and move them quickly to the bowl of ice water. Allow them to sit there for 2 minutes.

6. Crack the top of each of the egg and peel the shell away. Do this only at the tip.

7. When the wrapped asparagus are done, serve them with the runny egg as a dipping

Zesty Chicken Taco

Total Time	50 minutes	Fat	22g
Servings	4	Protein	30g
Calories per Serving	348	Carbs	5g

Ingredients for the tortilla filling:

1 whole lime

2 cups of lettuce

1 whole avocado

1 pound of chicken breast, boneless and skinless

Ingredients for the tortillas:

2 tablespoons of avocado oil

1/2 teaspoon of salt

1/4 cup of almond flour

1/4 cup of coconut flour

3/4 cup of egg whites

1/3 cup of water

Directions:

1. Preheat your oven to 400 degrees Fahrenheit.

2. Place a parchment paper over baking sheet. Arrange the chicken on the baking sheet. Bake for 35 minutes or until completely cooked.

3. Prepare the tortillas. Put all tortilla ingredients in a bowl. Mix them well, set aside and let it sit for 10 minutes.

4. Put the skillet over medium heat. Grease with avocado oil.

5. Pour 1/4 cup of batter into the skillet. Cook like a pancake. Cook the rest of the batter. And let them cool

6. Prepare the filling. Cut avocado and lime in half. Take the chicken out of the oven. Make pulled chicken.

7. Mix the chicken with the avocado flesh and lettuce. Squeeze lime over the filling. Stuff the cooled tortillas with the filling and serve.

Shrimp Stacks

Total Time	15 minutes	Fat	21.8g
Servings	4	Protein	12.3g
Calories per Serving	289	Carbs	14.2g

Ingredients:

1 teaspoon of pink salt

4 fresh basil leaves

2 whole limes

3 ripe avocados, pitted and diced

9 to 12 shrimps with tail on

coconut oil spray

Biscuit or cookie cutter

Directions:

1. Put a cooling rack on a sheet pan. Grease with coconut oil spray.

2. Place the shrimps on the grate. Season with salt. Spray with coconut oil.

3. Heat oven to 500 degrees Fahrenheit on Broil. Put the shrimp under the broiler for 5 minutes.

4. While waiting, mix avocado with lime juice, chopped basil, and salt.

5. Remove shrimp from heat.

6. Take a scoop of the avocado mixture and put into a cookie cutter. Fill up the circle and press down the plate. Slide the cookie cutter up to leave an avocado round. Place 3 to 4 shrimp on each of the avocado rounds with their tails up. Apply the same steps for the rest of the mixture and shrimps.

Crispy Bacon Wrapped Asparagus

Total Time	10 minutes	Fat	4g
Servings	12 bundles	Protein	3g
Calories per Serving	46 per bundle	Carbs	0g

Ingredients:

1 tablespoon of olive oil

12 slices of bacon

36 spears of asparagus

Salt and pepper

Directions:

1. Preheat your oven to 425. Use parchment paper to line baking sheet.

2. Take 3 asparagus spears and wrap with one bacon slice. Gently pull on the bacon as you wrap from bottom to top to ensure an even spiral layer. Do the same for the rest.

3. Arrange the wrapped asparagus on the baking sheet. Drizzle the bacon wrapped asparagus with olive oil. Season with salt and pepper.

4. Put inside the oven to bake for about 20 to 25 minutes or until the bacon is crispy.

Chapter 12 - FREQUENTLY ASKED QUESTIONS

How long until I reach ketosis?

You may reach ketosis anywhere from 2 to 7 days. The duration depends on several factors like your body type, your physical activity level as well as your current way of eating.

Can I have a cheat day?

Because you can get kicked out of ketosis easily and it would be difficult to regain progress, the ketogenic diet discourages cheat days or cheat meals.

Where do I find Low Carb Recipes?

Aside from those provided in this book, you can easily find keto-friendly recipes online. And when you do, make sure to look at the ingredients very closely.

How can I keep track if my carb intake?

Counting net carbs isn't rocket science. However, there are other quick ways to do it too. There are apps online that will help you monitor your carb consumption.

Is there a need to count calories?

Counting calories is not the focus of the ketogenic diet. It's hardly something you should be worried about. After all, fat and protein will keep you satiated for a longer time. If you do workout often, you may need to be mindful of your calorie intake but not obsess about it too much.

Can I eat too much fat?

As long as you are within your macro goals and calorie allowance goals, there's no need to worry about eating too much fat. You can try using a keto calculator which you will find conveniently online to help you make better decisions when it comes to macros.

How much weight will I be able to lose?

It all depends on how much and how long you stick to the diet. Initially, the weight loss can happen quickly because of water weight loss. For a more sustainable effect, you should not stray. Follow the rules and you will reach your weight loss goals.

Do I need to worry about having a heart attack from all the fat?

There are bad fat sources and good fat ones. The ketogenic diet emphasizes getting your fat from high-quality sources. If you seek and stick with the healthy fats, there's no need to worry.

What do I do, I feel like crap?

If you're just beginning with the diet, it is natural to feel the side effects. Your body is transitioning and the crappiness is natural. To feel less crappy, drink plenty of water and put salt in your food. Keto-friendly bacon and bone broth help a lot.

What do I do, I just stopped losing weight?

A weight loss plateau is a shared experience among weight loss watchers. Here are a couple of suggestions to help you from being stuck.

- Reduce dairy
- Increase your fat intake
- Decrease your carb intake further
- Stop eating gluten and nuts

- Let go of the sweeteners
- Check for hidden carbs

What happens when I stop eating ketosis?

When you stop the keto diet, your body will return to its usual routine of burning glucose for energy.

Can I work out while on Keto?

Exercise helps you burn fat. Ketosis does this for you. A lot of people lose weight on a ketogenic diet without lifting a finger but if you like the gym so much, you are free to do so too. A word of caution though. You may want to take it easy especially in the first few days or weeks of starting keto. Your body is still adjusting and you will feel some side effects. And moving forward, pay attention to your calorie intake. Since you're burning through ketosis and burning through exercise, you may need the extra help.

Can vegans/vegetarians do ketosis diet?

Yes. There are vegan options in a ketogenic diet.

What supplements do you recommend?

Among the most commonly recommended supplements include the following.

- Multivitamin for men and women
- Potassium supplement
- Magnesium supplement
- Vitamin D supplement
- Vitamin B complex

The safest way is to ask your doctor to prescribe vitamins and supplements that are right for you.

Conclusion

Congratulations! You've made it!

You now know more than you did before you picked this book up. I'm quite sure you're feeling challenged and excited to get on with it. Just remember though, ketosis is a process It is not something that you can choose on a whim. It's not something that you can get on and off anytime you like. Respect the process and you will be rewarded.

Are you ready to feel good?

Are you ready to get in shape?

Are you prepared for the challenges ahead?

Can you hardly wait for your best results?

Good luck and get on with it! May ketosis be with you!

SOURCES

Johnston, C. S., Day, C. S., & Swan, P. D. (2002). Postprandial thermogenesis is increased 100% on a high-protein, low-fat diet versus a high-carbohydrate, low-fat diet in healthy, young women. J Am Coll Nutr, 21(1), 55-61.

Ebbeling, C. B., Swain, J. F., Feldman, H. A., Wong, W. W., Hachey, D. L., Garcia-Lago, E., & Ludwig, D. S. (2012). Effects of dietary composition on energy expenditure during weight-loss maintenance. Jama, 307(24), 2627-2634.

Feinman, R. D., & Fine, E. J. (2004). "A calorie is a calorie" violates the second law of thermodynamics. Nutr J, 3, 9.

Bueno, N. B., de Melo, I. S., de Oliveira, S. L., & da Rocha Ataide, T. (2013). Very-low-carbohydrate ketogenic diet v. low-fat diet for long-term weight loss: a meta-analysis of randomised controlled trials. Br J Nutr, 110(7), 1178-1187.

Sackner-Bernstein, J., Kanter, D., & Kaul, S. (2015). Dietary Intervention for Overweight and Obese Adults: Comparison of Low-Carbohydrate and Low-Fat Diets. A Meta-Analysis. PLoS One, 10(10), e0139817.

Hallberg, S. J., McKenzie, A. L., Williams, P. T., Bhanpuri, N. H., Peters, A. L., Campbell, W. W., . . . Volek, J. S. (2018). Effectiveness and Safety of a Novel Care Model for the Management of Type 2 Diabetes at 1 Year: An Open-Label, Non-Randomized, Controlled Study. Diabetes Ther.

Volek, J.S., Sharman, M.J., Love, D.M., Avery, N.G., Gomez, A.L., Scheett, T.P., and Kraemer, W.J. (2002). Body composition and hormonal responses to a carbohydrate-restricted diet. Metabolism 51.

Paoli A, Rubini A, Volek JS, Grimaldi KA. Beyond weight loss: a review of the therapeutic uses of very-low-carbohydrate (ketogenic) diets. European Journal of Clinical Nutrition. 2013;67(8):789-796. doi:10.1038/ejcn.2013.116.

Gibson, A.A., Seimon, R.V., Lee, C.M., Ayre, J., Franklin, J., Markovic, T.P., Caterson, I.D., and Sainsbury, A. (2015). Do ketogenic diets really suppress appetite? A systematic review and meta-analysis. Obes. Rev. 16, 64-76.

Sumithran, P., Prendergast, L. A., Delbridge, E., Purcell, K., Shulkes, A., Kriketos, A., & Proietto, J. (2013). Ketosis and appetite-mediating nutrients and hormones after weight loss. Eur J Clin Nutr, 67(7), 759-764.

Johnstone, A. M., Horgan, G. W., Murison, S. D., Bremner, D. M., & Lobley, G. E. (2008). Effects of a high-protein ketogenic diet on hunger, appetite, and weight loss in obese men feeding ad libitum. Am J Clin Nutr, 87(1), 44-55.

Freeman, John M., et al. "The efficacy of the ketogenic diet— 1998: a prospective evaluation of intervention in 150 children." Pediatrics 102.6 (1998): 1358-1363.

Neal, Elizabeth G., et al. "The ketogenic diet for the treatment of childhood epilepsy: a randomised controlled trial." The Lancet Neurology 7.6 (2008): 500-506.

Yancy Jr, William S., et al. "A low-carbohydrate, ketogenic diet to treat type 2 diabetes." Nutr Metab (Lond) 2 (2005): 34.

Tóth C, Clemens Z. Type 1 diabetes mellitus successfully managed with the paleolithic ketogenic diet. Int J Case Rep Images 2014;5(10):699–703. http://www.ijcasereportsandimages.com/archive/2014/010-2014-ijcri/CR-10435-10-2014-clemens/ijcri-1043510201435-toth-full-text.php

Raised blood pressure. (2015, February 01). Retrieved from http://www.who.int/gho/ncd/risk_factors/blood_pressure_pr evalence_text/en/

Gardner, Christopher D., et al. "Comparison of the Atkins, Zone, Ornish, and LEARN diets for change in weight and related risk factors among overweight premenopausal women: The A TO Z Weight Loss Study: a randomized trial." Jama 297.9 (2007): 969-977.

Yancy, William S., et al. (2010). A randomized trial of a low-carbohydrate diet vs orlistat plus a low-fat diet for weight loss. Archives of internal medicine170.2 (2010): 136-145

Henderson S. T., Vogel J. L., Barr L. J., Garvin F., Jones J. J., Costantini L. C. (2009). Study of the ketogenic agent AC-1202 in mild to moderate Alzheimer's disease: a randomized, double-blind, placebo-controlled, multicenter trial. Nutr. Metab. (Lond.) 6, 31.10.1186/1743-7075-6-31

Vanitallie T. B., Nonas C., DiRocco A., Boyar K., Hyams K., Heymsfield S. B. (2005). Treatment of Parkinson disease with diet-induced hyperketonemia: a feasibility study. Neurology 64, 728–73010.1212/01.WNL.0000152046.11390.45, PubMed

Kim do Y., Vallejo J., Rho J. M. (2010). Ketones prevent synaptic dysfunction induced by mitochondrial respiratory complex inhibitors. J. Neurochem. 114, 130–141, PMC PubMed

Bueno, Nassib Bezerra, et al. "Very-low-carbohydrate ketogenic diet v. low-fat diet for long-term weight loss: a meta-analysis of randomised controlled trials." British Journal of Nutrition 110.07 (2013): 1178-1187.

Mavropoulos, J. C., Yancy, W. S., Hepburn, J., & Westman, E. C. (2005, December 16). The effects of a low-carbohydrate, ketogenic diet on the polycystic ovary syndrome: A pilot study.

Retrieved from
https://nutritionandmetabolism.biomedcentral.com/articles/1
0.1186/1743-7075-2-35

Tendler, D., Lin, S., Yancy Jr. W.S., Mavropoulos, J., Sylvestre,
P., Rockey, D.C., & Westman, E.C. (2007, January 12). The
Effect of a Low-Carbohydrate, Ketogenic Diet on Nonalcoholic
Fatty Liver Disease: A Pilot Study. Retrieved from
https://link.springer.com/article/10.1007/s10620-006-9433-5

Schwartz, K., Chang, H.T., Nikolai, M., Pernicone, J., Rhee, S.,
Olson, K., Kurniali, P.C., Hord, N.G., & Noel, M. (2015, March
25). Treatment of glioma patients with ketogenic diets: report
of two cases treated with an IRB-approved energy-restricted
ketogenic diet protocol and review of the literature. Retrieved
from
https://www.ncbi.nlm.nih.gov/pmc/articles/PMC4371612/

Di Lorenzo, C., Coppola, G., Sirianni, G., & Pierelli, F. (2013,
February 21). Short term improvement of migraine headaches
during ketogenic diet: a prospective observational study in a
dietician clinical setting. Retrieved from
https://www.ncbi.nlm.nih.gov/pmc/articles/PMC3620251/

Phinney, S.D. (2004, August 17). Ketogenic diets and physical
performance. Retrieved from
https://www.ncbi.nlm.nih.gov/pmc/articles/PMC524027/

Johnstone, A.M., Horgan, G.W., Murison, S.D., Bremner, D.M.,
& Lobley, G.E. (2008, January). Effects of a high-protein
ketogenic diet on hunger, appetite, and weight loss in obese
men feeding ad libitum. Retrieved from
https://www.ncbi.nlm.nih.gov/pubmed/18175736

Fernando, W.M., Martins, I.J., Goozee, K.G., Brennan, C.S.,
Jayasena, V., & Martins, R.N. (2015 July 14). The role of
dietary coconut for the prevention and treatment of

Alzheimer's disease: potential mechanisms of action. Retrieved from https://www.ncbi.nlm.nih.gov/pubmed/25997382

Nonaka, Y., Takagi, T., Inai, M., Nishimura, S., Urashima, S., Honda, K., Aoyama, T., & Terada, S. (2016 August 1). Lauric Acid Stimulates Ketone Body Production in the KT-5 Astrocyte Cell Line. Retrieved from https://www.ncbi.nlm.nih.gov/pubmed/27430387

Cox, P.J., & Clarke, K. (2014 October 29). Acute nutritional ketosis: implications for exercise performance and metabolism. Retrieved from https://www.ncbi.nlm.nih.gov/pubmed/25379174

Féry, F., & Balasse, E.O. (1986 May). Response of ketone body metabolism to exercise during transition from postabsorptive to fasted state. Retrieved from https://www.ncbi.nlm.nih.gov/pubmed/3518484

Borer, K.T., Wuorinen, E.C., Lukos, J.R., Denver, J.W., Porges, S.W., & Burant, C.F. (2009, August 4). Two bouts of exercise before meals, but not after meals, lower fasting blood glucose. Retrieved from https://www.ncbi.nlm.nih.gov/pubmed/19568199

Phinney, S.D. (2004 August 17). Ketogenic diets and physical performance. Retrieved from https://www.ncbi.nlm.nih.gov/pmc/articles/PMC524027/

Musa-Veloso, K., Likhodii, S.S., & Cunnane, S.C. (2002 July). Breath acetone is a reliable indicator of ketosis in adults consuming ketogenic meals. Retrieved from https://www.ncbi.nlm.nih.gov/pubmed/12081817

Wallace, T.M., Meston, N.M., Gardner, S.G., & Matthews, D.R. (2001, August). The hospital and home use of a 30-second hand-held blood ketone meter: guidelines for clinical practice. Retrieved from https://www.ncbi.nlm.nih.gov/pubmed/11553201